UROLOGY

UROLOGY
A VIEW THROUGH
THE RETROSPECTROSCOPE
JOHN R. HERMAN, M.D.

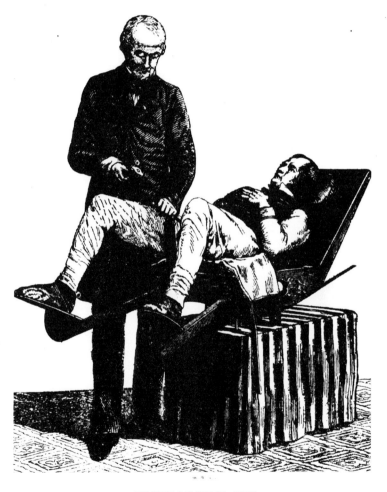

PUBLISHED BY
ACMI
STAMFORD, CONNECTICUT

Library of Congress Cataloging in Publication Data

Herman, John R.   1915–
    Urology, a view through the retrospectroscope.

    Bibliography: p.
    1. Urology—History.   I. Title.   [DNLM:
1. Urology—History.   WJ11 H551u 1973]
RC871.H448   616.6'009   73-11098
ISBN 0-06-141187-6

TO MY WIFE

who encouraged—and when necessary prodded and pushed—me. She it is who read, reread and finally proofread the manuscript and is now an expert in a field in which she had but little interest. Trite as it may be to say it, yet true for all of that: this work could not have been completed without her.

Contents

Preface

The adage "To understand the present you must know the past" holds particular relevance for me. To spend years in medical school, an internship and a residency, followed by many more years in practice, without knowing something about the background of the skills learned is, to me, incomprehensible. To be able to develop new techniques and methods and to fill in the gaps in our knowledge, it is indeed extremely helpful to "know the past."

A study of medical history need not be painful. For those who wish only to know the high points, a recital of dates and lists of strange-sounding names and places are tedious; they blunt—not whet —the appetite. Here then is offered a short description of the development of urology, to be read with ease and (hopefully) to be enjoyed. It should not be expected to serve either as a reference source or as a handbook for researchers in the field. Its aim is to impart some of the fascinating background of the oldest of the surgical specialties and consequently some of the early developments in medicine. If this work comes into the hands of medical students and residents and inculcates a sense of enjoyment of medical history, it will have served its purpose. If some of my professional colleagues then wish on their own to delve more deeply into the past—I welcome them to the field!

Publication of this work was made possible through the generous support and encouragement of the Bard Hospital Division of C. R.

Bard, Inc. I offer my sincere thanks for the help of many kind and patient people. Mr. Stanley Wayne and the members of the Audio-visual Department at the Albert Einstein College of Medicine provided most of the photographs. Mrs. Peggy Santonastaso and Mrs. Jacqueline Ingber typed and retyped the manuscript; their patience was boundless.

UROLOGY

The Beginnings

The penis is a sexy sewer and as such it has long been of interest to mankind. Indeed, since man has written interesting facts about himself, he has noted the rise and fall of the penis as a barometer of health. He has gazed intently at his urine, attempting to divine what was progressing inside his body. So, the genitourinary tract is discussed in the earliest medical records—the medical papyruses.

The Egyptian papyruses discovered in relatively modern times are thought to have been inscribed around 3000 B.C. They contain a body of medical knowledge that could not have sprung full-fledged from the Egyptians, but undoubtedly developed over many years and in many civilizations. The Hindus, Mohammedans, and perhaps the Chinese were advanced and well educated at these same times, and they also were developing a wealth of medical knowledge. Their early writings either are nonexistent or have not yet been discovered.

The Egyptian papyruses that have been salvaged and translated are generally known after the names of the Egyptologists who located or translated them. It is a common tendency to shrug off the Egyptian papyruses and their hieroglyphics as too complicated and too difficult to be of interest. However, a careful examination of the pages of the papyrus in the New York Academy of Medicine Library reveals certain hieroglyphic figures of interest to urologists. Perhaps the most interesting of these figures is that of a penis and testes. With small waving lines under it, the figure signifying the male genitals becomes the figure for urine (line 14, Fig. 1). These are seen in the hieroglyphic transliteration of the papyrus. In

the originals they are lines drawn to indicate the same, as

$\wedge$ ⌐ or $\wedge$ ≋ . Some are even shown as $\wedge$ ⌐ ⟩

transliterated to ⌒ ⌒≋ . Other pictures are quite

obviously fish, people, and animals.

The Edwin Smith Papyrus refers to case histories and gives therapies and prognoses. Case 31 is translated as follows.*

If thou examinest a man having a dislocation in a vertebra of his neck, shouldst thou find him unconscious of his two arms [and] his two legs on account of it, while his phallus is erected on account of it, [and] urine drops from his member without his knowing of it; his flesh has received wind; his two eyes are blood-shot; it is a dislocation of a vertebra of his neck extending to his backbone which causes him to be unconscious of his two arms and legs. If, however, the middle vertebra of his neck is dislocated, it is an emissio seminis which befalls his phallus.

This is a pretty acute observation made 5000 years ago. This papyrus, incidentally, is held by the library of the New York Academy of Medicine, where it may be viewed by anyone so desiring. It looks as if it had been written yesterday.

The Ebers Papyrus refers to retention, incontinence, cystitis, prostatitis, and urethritis. It especially refers to hematuria, suggesting that it is caused by parasites. Bilharzial disease was

* Breasted JH: *The Edwin Smith Surgical Papyrus,* Vol. XI. University of Chicago Press, 1930.

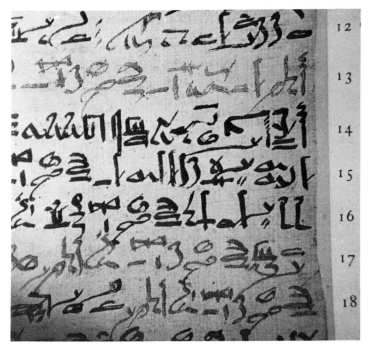

FIG. 1. *Photographs of papyrus. (From Breasted JH: The Edwin Smith Surgical Papyrus. vol XI, University of Chicago Press, 1930.)*

known to the Egyptians, and it is said that probably because of this, a leather or bark codpiece was worn on the penis to prevent the parasites from going up the urethra into the bladder. Interestingly, modern explorers have found Indian tribes in upper remote regions of the Amazon River wearing almost identical codpieces. However, these are worn to prevent the Candiru, a catfish, from gaining access to the urethra.

It is difficult to understand why the Egyptians, advanced in medical and scientific knowledge as they were, would wear a codpiece to prevent bilharzial infestation, which of course does not occur via the urethra. They must have been aware of this, and although it has not yet been proved, we might presume that some urophilic parasites existed in the Nile valley. Such parasitism could parallel the dangers encountered by the Amazon tribes whose members wear codpieces to prevent urethral invasion by the Candiru, the only known vertebrate parasite of man. History is still being rediscovered.

The Egyptians wrote of vesical calculi, bilharzial stones, dysuria, incontinence, retention, and enuresis. They often prescribed urine for medication. They also utilized what we scornfully refer to as "sewage pharmacology." Fly droppings, feces, gazelle dung, crocodile excrement, mud from burial grounds, and mouldy bread were all used. Modern science has recovered penicillin from bread moulds, and Aureomycin was originally recovered from soil found near cemeteries.

Circumcision is depicted on the walls of a building thought to be a temple. It was done at the age of 10 to 12, but only on special youths. Although Egyptians did circumcision and brain surgery, they also believed in incantations and prayers as a part of therapy. They used reeds, bronze and tin catheters, and sounds to relieve obstructions. Juniper berries (from which gin is made) were used for a diuretic, and beer was often a vehicle for medications of the genitourinary tract. Medications were offered for both excessive urination and discharge of small quantities of urine.

Stones were well known and, indeed, one of the earliest uroliths recovered was found in the nasal cavity of a mummy. It obviously was forgotten in replacing the viscera and placed there as a last resort. What was probably the chronologically earliest calculus yet discovered was destroyed in an English museum during the London Blitz.

The Hindu civilization also goes back centuries. The Hindus, rather than writing about or depicting their civilization on papyrus or stones, composed major monumental poems or stories known as *Vedas* or *Samhitas*. These were memorized and passed down through the generations. Not only are their dates and origins unknown, but also the final written versions may differ markedly from the earlier unwritten stories. However, what we do know is that these Vedas and Samhitas reflect an advanced knowledge of medicine and surgery. The description of the surgical procedure for vesical calculus was carefully detailed:*

The patient should be soothed by the application of oleaginous substances, his system should be cleansed with emetics and purgatives and be slightly reduced thereby. . . . Prayers, offerings and prophylactic charms should be offered and the instruments and surgical accessories required in this case should be arranged. . . . The surgeon should use his best endeavors to encourage the patient and infuse hope and courage in the patient's mind. . . . [The manner of securing the patient on the table is then detailed—ed.] After that the umbilical region of the patient should be well rubbed with oil or clarified butter and the left side of the abdomen pressed with a closed fist so that the stone comes within reach of the operator. The surgeon should then introduce into the rectum the second and third fingers of his left hand, duly anointed and with nails well pared. Then the fingers should be carried upward . . . to bring the stone between the rectum and the penis, when it should be so firmly and strongly pressed as to look like an elevated tumor. An incision should then be made on the left side of the raphe of the perineum at the distance of a barley corn and of a sufficient width to allow the free egress of the stone.

Postoperative care includes:

The patient should be made to sit in a cauldron full of warm water . . . in doing so the possibility of an accumulation of blood in the bladder will be prevented. . . . However if blood be accumulated therein, a decoction should be injected into the bladder with the help of a urethral syringe.

Remember, these postoperative orders were not dictated last year, but probably 4000 to 5000 years ago. The *Sushruta Samhita* even reminds us not to leave any pieces of the stone behind, "as they would in such case be sure to grow larger again." The knowledge of urolithogenesis was indeed well

* Bhishagratna KL: *An English Translation of the Sushruta Samhita.* Varanasi, Chowkhamba Sanskrit Series Office, 1963.

advanced in this period, but the surgeon was warned in advance:

Surgical operations in these cases do not prove successful even in the hands of a skillful and experienced surgeon, so lithotomic operations should be considered a remedy that has little to recommend itself. The death of the patient is almost certain without a surgical operation and the result to be derived from it is also uncertain.

Mesopotamian medicine also was advanced and it nearly paralleled that of Egypt chronologically. Both countries entered the period of written history about 3000 B.C. The earliest historians—the Sumerians—impressed their cuneiform writings on soft clay, and it is from these that we have learned of the urology of the period. Gonorrhea was known as follows: "If a man's urine is like the urine of an ass, that man is sick of gonorrhea; if a man's urine is like beer yeast, that man is sick of gonorrhea; if a man's urine is like gummy varnish, that man is sick of gonorrhea."* Discharges of pus or blood, spermatorrhea, retention of urine, incontinence of urine, impotence, and related subjects are discussed; remedies include prescriptions and general love charms.

Impotence and the use of aphrodisiacs made up an important part of the early practitioner's work load. The *Sushruta Samhita* gives considerable space to the discussion of aphrodisiacs, or Vaji-Karana, described as follows:†

If duly taken, these remedies make a man sexually as strong as a horse and enable him to cheerfully satisfy the heat and amorous ardours of young maidens. . . . Old men, those wishing to enjoy sexual pleasures or to secure the affection of women, as well as those suffering from senile decay or sexual incapacity, and persons

* Sigerist Henry E: *A History of Medicine,* Vol I: Primitive and Archaic Medicine (From Thompson RC: Assyrian prescriptions for diseases of the urine. *Babylonaica,* Vol XIV, 1934.) New York, Oxford University Press, 1955.

† Bhishagratna KL: *An English Translation of the Sushruta Samhita.* Varanasi, Chowkhamba Sanskrit Series Office, 1963.

weakened with sexual excesses should do well to submit themselves to a course of these remedies.

The first description of aphrodisiacs might have been reproduced from Playboy magazine:

Various kinds of food, liquid cordials, speech that gladdens the ears and touch which seems delicious to the skin, clear nights mellowed by the beams of the full moon and damsels young and beautiful, wine and flowers and a merry, careless heart, these are the best aphrodisiacs.

In spite of these natural methods, various substances are mixed and prescribed in order that "a man would be able to visit a hundred women"; a man becomes potent enough to enjoy "the pleasures of love, like a sparrow"; and "this compound would make even an old man of eighty sexually as vigorous as a youth." Finally, by lubricating the soles of his feet with one such mixture, "a man would be able to visit a woman with undiminished vigour so long as he would not touch the ground with his feet."

The Hindu writings record a tremendous body of knowledge of stone and urinary obstructions. The "lithologists" were the first specialists, and they were a proud group. There were rules for their behavior and plans for their education were complex. When considered ready for the practice of lithology, they were told to try out their lithologic skills on three heretics: "If these all die, practice no more, for if you do and the man dies, it is murder."

The *Ayurveda* of Sushruta suggested, among many other things, that malaria was caused by mosquitoes, that there was a honey urine disease (diabetes), that *Cannabis indica* could be used for analgesia. Sounds, catheters, and bougies were described and student practitioners were taught to tap hydroceles by practicing on gourds.

Urology was multicentric in origin. In addition to the Hindus and the Egyptians, the Chinese were also developing a large body of medical knowledge. By 1100 BC, socialized

medicine was being practiced in China. The state had examinations for doctors, and salaries were allotted on the basis of
work estimated for the year. They developed theories and
philosophies of medicine that were the basis for some of the
therapies. The Chinese thought that:*

> *Liver stores the blood and controls the soul.*
> *Heart controls the pulse and the spirit.*
> *Spleen stores nutrition and controls ideas or thoughts.*
> *The kidney controls the spittle, the bones and the will.*

Each organ had a color, a taste, a season, a parent, and
enemies. Thus, the heart was the son of the liver, friend of the
spleen, and its enemy was the kidney. Harry Goldblatt, several
thousand years later, found that the kidney with vascular
disease is indeed a danger to the heart. Interestingly, the only
surgical procedure mentioned is castration. The Chinese felt
that surgery was an admission of the failure of medicine. The
Central American Olmecs, antecedents of the Aztecs, used
sarsaparilla as a diuretic. To increase sexual potency they
advised the taking of colorimes—a seed—to stimulate the erection center in the spinal cord. They, too, were burdened with
the inevitable problems of impotency.

Circumcision, often called the first elective surgery (though
often connected with religion), was also multicentric in origin. Just as man's worship of the supernatural probably resulted from insecurity and fear brought on by his strange
contacts with life and death and other natural phenomena, so
he was mystified by fertility and reproduction. He hoped that
rituals and magic might help influence these natural phenomena.

Animal and human sacrifices were required in some areas,
but eventually the letting of human blood was sufficient. This
was usually done by incising the infants' foreskin. In other

* VEITH ILZA (trans): *HUANG TI NEI CHING SU WÊN,* The
Yellow Emperor's Classic of Internal Medicine. Berkeley, University of
California Press, 1966.

regions and tribal groups, circumcision was carried out to mark the passage of youth into manhood. Some of the early Arabian tribes routinely circumcised men on their wedding day. This rough, painful, unsterile surgery often resulted in mutilation and death. If the male flinched or showed the slightest sign of pain, the bride-to-be might refuse to marry him. If the marriage was accepted, certainly there was no need for birth control measures for the first part of the honeymoon.

In addition to the magic, religious, and tribal rites there may well have been physiologic reasons for circumcision among the pubertal boys, readying them for coitus. If the prepuce was overly long, could not be retracted, or was thickened, infected, or contained foreign bodies, then circumcision was needed before sexual activity began. However, in view of our modern findings, this could only have been a factor in a small percentage of lads.

Egyptians, Amorites, Hittites, and others had all been practicing circumcision when Abraham made his convenant with God for the Jews. Abraham was told: ". . . an uncircumcised male who does not circumcise the flesh of his foreskin shall be cut off from his kin." (Genesis 17:11). Jews were told in Leviticus 12:3 to circumcise their boys on the eighth day after birth. Therefore, the surgical procedure became a religious procedure again, and the cycle had been completed.

The Bible has other urologic references that might be carefully noted. In Leviticus 15:3 it is stated: "When a man has a discharge issuing from his member, he is unclean." In other passages, it was made fairly definite that when he becomes clean of his discharge, "he shall count off seven days for his cleansing, wash his clothes, and bathe his body with fresh water; then he shall be clean." (Leviticus 15:13.)

Reviewing the years from the times of the early Egyptian pharaohs, the Hindu Vedas, the Chinese writings, and the other early histories, we can only pick out here and there an outstanding name whose fame has lasted through the ages. Urology has been, of course, the major thrust of medicine for many of the years of recorded history, and has been in the forefront well into modern times. Outstanding names in medicine must, of necessity, have been important names in urology. All the important names can't be mentioned, but skipping here and there we shall see how urology and uroscopy have developed.

Uroscopy was the art of looking into a glass container of urine and being able to diagnose the patient's condition and prescribe a course of therapy without necessarily seeing the patient at all. Uroscopy was a natural development of man's curiosity about himself. After all, urine is the most readily examined of the body's outputs. It varies greatly with intake, with the state of the body, and specifically with affectations of the urinary tract. To be able to examine the urine, diagnose, and prescribe seemed to border on magic, and this was done frequently by friends or clients. Uroscopists ran the gamut from highly respected professionals to fly-by-night mountebanks.

Such highly respected men of medicine as Hippocrates (460–377 BC) made much of examination of the urine. His book of uroscopy was widely accepted as gospel. Hippocrates absorbed some of his knowledge from the Egyptians and the Hindus; indeed, he was very widely educated. Realizing the importance of the urine in reflecting the state of the body, he suggested nephrotomy for suppuration of the kidney (thought to be due to stone and obstruction) . This was not accepted for many years, although perirenal abscesses were opened not too many years later. He placed a very vigorous veto on cutting into the bladder suprapubically. Hippocrates was also said to be the originator of that now inappropriate famous oath: "I will not use the knife even on sufferers from stone, but will give place to those who are craftsmen therein."

Going back to uroscopy, the Hindus let fall a drop of oil into a urine sample and based on its floating, sinking or spreading prognosticated the patient's condition. The Chinese *Nei-Ching* (The Yellow Emperor's Classic of Internal Medicine) describes urine and how it differs with disease. Others wrote of the smell of urine, the taste of urine (still advised into the sixteenth and seventeenth centuries), the color of urine, and its clarity or cloudiness. Artists of the period picked the subject of the doctor or uroscopist and the typical urine sample bottles for many now-famous paintings. The urine sample was usually carried in a matula, a glass container, bulbous at the bottom and funnel-shaped above a relatively narrow waist. This matula was usually transported in a wicker basket with a top; so many of the paintings show these familiar containers and medical doctors or uroscopists examining the urine. From foretelling or diagnosing pregnancy to predicting the sex of an unborn baby, the uroscopists attempted to learn much more than was actually indicated from the urine bubbles, granules, opacities, pus, fat, sand, ash, and other sediment, as well as from the smell, sound, taste, and amount of urine. Often the forecast depended on what the uroscopist could learn from the messenger who brought the specimen. Honest uroscopists also existed, and they advanced the study of urine.

Hippocrates recognized at least hematuria, lithiasis (colic), suppuration, and probably tuberculosis. Aretaeus the Cappadocian, living in the second century of the Christian era, wrote of how to distinguish acute from chronic nephritis by the urine, among other things. Rufus of Ephesus, in Trajan's reign, attempted to differentiate between vesical and renal hematuria.

Aetius, a Mesopotamian doctor about 500 AD, wrote a systemic classification of urinalysis. He was followed by Alexander of Tralles in the sixth century and Theophilus in the seventh century writing treatises of urinologic diagnosis. Thereafter uroscopy was an important method of diagnosing disease until 1694. In that year, Frederik Dekkers, by boiling urine from a "sick" kidney, discovered and realized some of the significance of albuminuria. The old joke about the man who, after an analysis of a urine sample, went home and said to his daughter, his wife, and his sister: "one of you is pregnant"—may well have originated before the time of Christ.

The basic knowledge of urinary physiology, which finally led medicine to its present position, was known very early in history. Aretaeus the Cappadocian is reported to have written of the bladder:*

But, also, its office is of vital importance; namely, the passage of the urine. Even, then, when the passage is only stopped by stones, or clots, or from any native or foreign mischief, it is of a deadly nature. In many cases, too, owing to involuntary restraint from modesty in assemblies and at banquets, being filled, it becomes distended; and, from the loss of its contractile power, it no longer evacuates the urine. When the urine is stopped, there is fullness of the parts above, namely the kidneys, distention of the ureters, grievous pain of the loins, spasms, tremblings, rigors, alienation of the mind.

This sounds like a description from modern times.

Before the birth of Christ, urologic surgery was progressing in the field of urolithiasis. Herophilus of Chalcedonia (about 400 BC) was a lithologist whose perineal incisions must have been high, wide and fancy. He was able to describe the prostate gland and also what were probably the seminal vesicles. Celsus, only a few years later, performed urethrotomy for impacted urethral calculus. Remember, this was still before the birth of Christ.

The first outstanding physician after Christ was the Roman Claudius Galen, a giant of his time. Physician to the gladiators, anatomy demonstrator at the medical school, researcher, —he was a writer of articles and many books and practitioner of the art and science of medicine, not unlike the typical modern "volunteer attending." He wrote of incontinence and retention, and described the S-shaped catheter. His books dominated medicine for years and influenced the practice of physicians probably for centuries. He wrote of the passage of urine from the kidneys through the ureters to the bladder, a natural course of events accepted without thought now, but argued strenuously by Asklepiades and his school. Galen proved his point without difficulty in a still living cow.

* *The Extant Works of Aretaeus, The Cappadocian.* Printed for the Sydenham Society, Wertheimer Co., London, Finsbury Circus, 1856.

Remember, the year was about 170 AD; not till 209 AD did the Romans conquer Britain. A sample of his writings may do much to demonstrate the strength and character of the man who was Claudius Galen.*

Failure of Asklepiades to Understand the Function of the Kidneys and Ureters

The extent of exactitude and truth in the doctrines of Hippocrates may be gauged, not merely from the way in which his opponents are at variance with obvious facts, but also from the various subjects of natural research themselves—the functions of animals and the rest. For those people, who do not believe that there exists in any part of the animal a faculty for attracting its own special quality, are compelled repeatedly to deny obvious facts. For instance, Asklepiades, the physician, did this in the case of the kidneys. That these are organs for secreting the urine was the belief not only of Hippocrates, Diocles, Erasistratos, Praxagoras, and all other physicians of eminence, but practically every butcher is aware of this, from the fact that he daily observes both the position of the kidneys and the duct, or ureter, which runs from each kidney into the bladder, and from this arrangement he infers their characteristic use and faculty. But, even leaving the butchers aside, all people who suffer either frequent dysuria, or from retention of the urine, call themselves "nephritics" when they feel pain in the loins and pass sandy matter in their water.

I do not suppose that Asklepiades ever saw a stone which had been passed by one of these sufferers, or observed that this was preceded by a sharp pain in the region between kidneys and bladder, as the stone traversed the ureter, or that, when the stone was passed, both the pain and the retention at once ceased. It is worth while, then, learning how his theory accounts for the presence of urine in the bladder and one is forced to marvel at the ingenuity of a man who puts aside these broad, clearly visible routes, and postulates others, which are narrow, invisible, indeed, entirely imperceptible. His view, in fact, is that the fluid which we drink, passes into

* Selwyn-Brown Arthur: *The Physician Throughout the Ages.* Vol I, New York, Capehart Brown Co., 1938.

the bladder by being resolved into vapors and that, when these again have been condensed, it thus regains its previous form, and turns from vapor into fluid. He simply looks upon the bladder as a sponge, or a piece of wool, and not as the perfectly compact and impervious body that it is, with two very strong coats. For, if we say that the vapors pass through these coats, why should they not pass through the peritoneum and the diaphragm, thus filling the whole abdominal cavity and thorax with water? "But," says he, "of course the peritoneal coat is more impervious than the bladder, and this is why it keeps out the vapors, while the bladder admits them." Yet, if he had ever practiced anatomy, he might have known that the outer coat of the bladder springs from the peritoneum and is essentially the same as it, and that the inner coat, which is peculiar to the bladder, is more than twice as thick as the former.

Perhaps it is not the thickness or thinness of the coats, but the situation of the bladder, which is the reason for the vapors being carried with it? On the contrary, even if it were probable for every other reason that the vapors accumulate there, yet the situation of the bladder would be enough in itself to prevent this. For the bladder is situated below, whereas vapors have a tendency to rise upwards; thus they would fill all the region of the thorax and lungs long before they reached the bladder.

But why do I mention the situation of the bladder, peritoneum, and thorax? For surely, when the vapors have passed through the coats of the stomach and intestines, it is in the space between these and the peritoneum that most of the water gathers. Otherwise the vapors must necessarily pass straight forward through everything which in any way comes in contact with them, and will never come to a standstill. But if this is assumed, then they will traverse not merely the peritoneum but also the epigastrium, and will become dispersed into the surrounding air; otherwise they will certainly collect under the skin.

Even these considerations, however, our present-day Asklepiadeans attempt to answer, despite the fact that they always get soundly laughed at by all who happen to be present at their lectures on these subjects—so difficult an evil to rid of is this sectarian partisanship, so excessively resistant to all cleansing processes, harder to heal than an itch.

Thus, one of our Sophists who is a thoroughly hardened disputer, and as skillful a master of language as there ever was, once got into a discussion with me on the subject. So far from being put out of countenance by any of the above mentioned considerations, he even expressed surprise that I should try to overturn obvious facts by ridiculous arguments.

"For," said he, "one may clearly observe any date in the case of any bladder, that, if one fills it with water or air and then ties up its neck and squeezes it all around, it does not let anything out at any point, but accurately contains all its contents. And surely, if there were any large and perceptible channels coming into it from the kidneys, the liquid would run out through these when the bladder is squeezed, in the same way that it entered."

Having abruptly made these and similar remarks in precise and clear tones, he concluded by jumping up and departing, leaving me as though I were quite incapable of finding any plausible answer.

We were, therefore, to show how the urine flows, in a still living animal.

Galen's description of the reproductive apparatus deserves repetition here. It is a contrast of detailed knowledge and complete lack of information:*

The reproductive apparatus is composed in man of testicles, placed out of the body, in the scrotum, sanguineous vessels, and nerves; the epididymus, a small body placed on the upper part of the testicles; the spermatic canal, or vas deferens; the vesiculae seminalae, the prostate gland; and the penis, which is a nervous and hollow body, springing from the ossa pubis, but containing no humor. In women, whose nature is colder than that of man, the sexual parts are placed in the interior of the body. The testicles, which are smaller, are situated on the sides of the uterus, and within the abdomen. The spermatic ducts (uterine tubes) unite the testicles to the uterus, which is placed between the bladder and the rectum. Galen speaks of two uterine cavities, one on the right, destined for the male fetus, the other on the left, for the female. . . . In coition the semen of the male, which is hotter than that of the female, mingles with the latter, which serves as an excipient and nutritive material; from this results fecundation. The semen changes at first into membranes,

* Renouard PV: *History of Medicine.* Translated by Cornelius G Comegys, MD, Philadelphia, Lindsay & Blakiston, 1867.

then a portion of these are transformed into cartilages and bones; another portion is folded and hollowed, and extends itself in the form of pipes, which constitute the arteries and veins.

The word artery comes from the Greek and means air duct. They may have been so called because arteries examined after death were often found to be filled with gas or air. Aretaeus the Cappadocian probably lived shortly after Galen, although he never mentioned Galen in his writings. He, too, was a prolific writer and discussed many topics of interest to urologists. His writings included descriptions of acute affections of the kidney, chronic affections of the kidney, acute affections of or about the bladder, chronic affections of the bladder, gonorrhea and colic. He also discusses the cures for these conditions.

Most of his discussion of acute kidney disease is of stones and the obstructions they cause and the "dreadful symptoms" produced by the retention of urine: "acrid heat, nausea, a heavy pain in the loin, distention of the parts, suppression of urine, not entirely, but they pass urine in drops, and have a desire to pass more, for there is the sensation of an overflow."

Aretaeus further describes uremia:*

Pulse, at first, indeed slow and languid; but, if the evil press harder, small, frequent, tumultuous and irregular; sleep slight, painful, not continued and suddenly starting up as if from the stroke of a sharp instrument, they fall over again into a deep sleep as if from fatigue. They are not deranged in intellect, but talk incoherently; the countenance livid. Of those that die, they sink most quickly who pass no urine; but the greater part recover, either from the stone dropping down into the bladder along with the urine, or from the inflammation being converted into pus or from being gradually dispelled.

Most interesting to urologists is the description by Aretaeus of acute and chronic nephritis:

* *The Extant Works of Aretaeus, the Cappadocian.* Translated by Francis Adams. London, Printed for the Sydenham Society, Wertheimer Co., Finsburg Circus, 1856.

Sometimes blood bursts from the kidneys suddenly in large quantity and flows continuously for many days. None, however, die from the hemorrhage itself, but from the inflammation accompanying the hemorrhage, if the bleeding is stopped; but most frequently they die of strong inflammation induced by the stoppage.

His description of chronic nephritis must strike a note of familiarity:

Certain persons pass bloody urine periodically: This affection resembles that from hemorrhoids, and the constitution of the body is alike; they are very pale, inert, sluggish without appetite, without digestion, and if the discharge has taken place, they are languid and relaxed in their limbs, but light and agile in their head. But if the periodical evacuation do not take place, they are afflicted with headache, their eyes become dim, dull and rolling, hence many become epileptic; others are swollen, musty, dropsical, and others again are affected with melancholy and paralysis.

This description would easily depict some of the present-day nephrotics. Aretaeus was an acute clinician and his writings reflect his observations. Many were the practitioners who described instruments for the removal or diagnosis of stones, or for new ways of diagnosis by uroscopy. However, through the fall of the Holy Roman Empire, the middle ages, and into the feudal ages, there were few outstanding advances. The monks controlled most of medicine, and generally they wanted little to do with the surgical approaches to disease.

Books were written describing uroscopic findings. Paroxysmal hemoglobinuria was ascribed to exposure to cold by Actuarius of Byzantium, and Peter Carbolensis in 1140 wrote *Liber di Urinus,* a classification of diseases by uroscopic findings. These were evaluated in a carefully regulated manner as follows: The urine was first collected in a transparent urine container and examined in respect to four main aspects: color, concentration, quantity, and contents. Even the sound made by a sliver of wood hitting the surface was an aid in diagnosis. Incidentally, color charts were available for comparing urine colors and about twenty different shades were recognized. Depending on which school of uroscopy one followed, the urine in the glass was divided. In one school, the portion called the Circulus indicated diseases of the head; Superfices, diseases of the breast; Perferatio, diseases of the stomach; and Fundus, diseases of the urinary organs. In other words, changes from the normal in those portions pointed to pathology in these organ systems. Another school merely divided the urine into four layers, and to each gave special significance. These layers were logically enough the Superfices, or surface; the Nubes, or uppermost layer; the Sublima, or middle layer; and the Hypostases, or lowermost part. Special note was made of the content of bubbles, granules of different colors, opacities, pus, fat, blood, sand, stones, atoms, and sediment.

In *Grounds of Physick,* John Greenfield, M.D., "a Member of the College of Physicians," wrote many years later:*

Here we speak of urine only as it is an Effect, which points out some Cause in some part of the Body. So it denotes to us the Temper of the Body, or something particular concerning its parts, which the Serum continually passes through; as it is from them that it is varyed in its Colour, Substance, or Quality. But that we may learn the most from the Inspection of the Urine, it ought to be that which is made after Chilification is finished, whether it be in Night or Day Time.

Grounds of Physick is written in dialogue form, and the next few questions and answers are very interesting and revealing:

Q. "How is the Urine of a Brute known from that of a Man?"
A. "If on purpose to deceive, such Urine is shewed for a Mans, the best way to know it is from its smell."

----

* Greenfield John: *Grounds of Physick,* containing so much of Philosophy, Anatomy, Chimistry, and *the Mechanical Construction of a Humane Body, as is necessary to the Accomplishment of a Physitian; With the Method of Practice in Common Distempers. London,* Printed by J Dover for W Taylor in Paternoster-Row, J Osborn in Lombard Street, and J Pemberton, in Fleet-Street, 1715.

Q. "What things are chiefly known from the Urine?"

A. "Chiefly the good or bad Constitution of those parts from whence the Urine has its Generation and Perfection. Hence, when we see different Colours of Urine, it is a diagnostick of Life or Death, as we shall see in what follows."

Q. "But does not urine instruct us upon various Accounts?"

A. "It is to be considered variously, as upon account of Colour, Smell, Taste, Quantity, Consistance, and several other of its Contents, frequently observable therein."

The next chapters of this book are concerned with the "Colour of Urine" and its causes, and then next "Of the Smell and Taste of Urine." Here we learn that urine has a naturally "Stinking, Strong, and Sulphureous" odor, or if it ". . . wants smell, it denotes too hasty a secretion."

Q. "Is it within the physician's dignity to taste the urine?"

A. "No, that shall be done by the patient or the patient's servant and reported to the physician, and if that cannot be done, the physician had better inquire nothing about it."

This remarkable book then deals with the "Consistance of Urine" and we learn there are four kinds of "distempered urine." The first is too thick, the second is turbid, the third is thin, and the fourth is transparent urine. The questioner here attempts to clarify the last:

Q. "How comes the Urine to be transparent?"

A. "The Fourth, is transparent Urine; when there is less gross Matter between the serous Particles of the Urine, so that the Rays of Light are more easily and more directly transmitted."

Q. "What is the cause of muddy Urine?"

A. "A cause contrary to the former."

And the last chapter on urine deals with its contents, stating "it is something visible in the substance of the urine" under two groupings: Universal and Particular. The Universal is common almost to all urines, and is threefold: the Hypostasis, or that which settles to the bottom; the Eneorema, that which is suspended in the middle; and the Nubecula, or little cloud that floats near the top! This is discussed further in Chapter 16, Urinalysis.

Columbus is said to have discovered the Americas in 1492, and this is the approximate date given by many for the introduction of syphilis on the European continent. In China, syphilis is thought to go back to the Ming Dynasty (1368–1644). According to some researchers into medical history, syphilis was known in Europe long before the time of Columbus. Professor Karl Sudhoff believed syphilis was extant, although known by several different names, early in the twelfth century. Mercurial inunctions certainly have been known, described, and used since those days, mostly for an "indefinable group of skin eruptions." Those yielding to mercurial inunctions were spirochetal and probably syphilis. Mercurial salves have been widely used in many countries and Sudhoff believed that syphilis was endemic in Italy as early as 1429.

These are, of course, only indirect proofs and the story that Columbus' sailors introduced syphilis will probably long retain its flavor. Flavor is also added to this history if we accept the story that in 1495, at the siege of Naples by France, syphilis was thought to be rampant. The French, of course, picked up the disease from the Spanish occupants who had picked it up from Columbus' sailors. It was then called the French or Spanish pox, the Polish pox, the German, Turkish or Italian pox, as each country attempted to pass the "honors" on to another as originator of the scourge known as syphilis. The king's pox and the French pox seem to have been favorite terms used to describe it.

Although mercurial ointments were known and used for years before Columbus' famous trip, syphilis and its venereal origins were not understood until about 1500. Astrologists are said to have prognosticated the approach of a venereal disease; others thought the disease due to floods, to intercourse of a leper with a prostitute, to the poisoning of water supplies, or to eating disguised human flesh. Its venereal nature was quickly recognized after it became pandemic and began to spread north and south from Italy. It rapidly proved the rule that a disease is no respecter of persons as it spread among all classes in all civilizations.

During the Renaissance came the revival of learning and the restoration of education. The use of gunpowder in Europe, the invention of printing, and the enlargement of the world by the discoveries of Columbus, Vasco da Gama, and Magellan all stimulated thought and opened new fields of endeavor. With these new and critical thoughts came new approaches to medicine. The writings of Hippocrates and Galen were set in print and circulated for the educated. Interestingly enough, spectacles—invented two centuries earlier—came into general use only after printing became widespread. Doctors lectured in medical schools, using Greek and Latin texts of the great masters as the basis for their discussions. No longer were "facts" accepted uncritically, but each was tested as far as possible before it was accepted. The atmosphere of the times must have strongly resembled the present upsurge of the "questioning approach." No longer was what was good enough for dad, good enough for son. Each new group searched its own way. The foundation of education, then as now, became the teaching of how to learn—not the teaching of facts, but how to find one's own facts. This, then, was the Renaissance, the rebirth of the search for knowledge. Its effect on medicine was enormous.

Lithotomy
or "Cutting for Stone"

Just prior to the Renaissance, lithologists had formed a recognized and licensed guild that stood high in rank with others, just below the fur skinners guild. They had a strict rule of order and were penalized if their work was not satisfactory. They were tested by operating on convicted criminals. If the criminal lived, he was usually pardoned and the surgeon "licensed" to "operate for gain." If he died or the operation failed, the prospective surgeon "failed his boards," but could be examined elsewhere at a later date. New operative procedures which had reached levels wherein the "establishment" thought they might have merit, were also tried out on criminals. In 1475, Colot thought that it would be cleaner, easier, and less likely to cause permanent damage if he could remove stones suprapubically. He persuaded the establishment and his peers, and he was given a criminal on whom to try out his operation. The operation—an abdominal approach to the bladder—was successful; the criminal lived. However, Colot's peers, perhaps still intimidated by Hippocrates' mandate that it was too dangerous, found it unsafe. The suprapubic approach to the bladder was thus forgotten for many years until the time of John Douglas, brother of the anatomist whose name has been attached to the peritoneal pouch in the pelvis. More of this later.

Lithotomy was divided into two different operations at this time. The "apparatus minor," or lesser operation, was the time-honored operation of pushing the stone into the perineum with the fingers in the rectum and then cutting down directly on the protruding lump caused by the stone. The instruments needed for this procedure were a knife or knives, a hook, and a forceps of sorts to remove the stone (Fig. 2).

The operation was accomplished in a very short time. As a matter of fact, the lithotomists were often timed by the bystanders, and many did the entire procedure in two minutes or less. Their knives were wrapped with linens at the proper depth, so that the stabbing incisions would not penetrate too deeply. The operation was a brutal manhandling of tissues with little or no regard for anatomy. It was not very readily used for adult males because the prostate got in the way.

In 1520, John de Romani (also called Francisco Romano), surgeon of Cremona, suggested the "apparatus major." This required more instruments and was a more anatomic procedure. Mariano Santo de Barletta, one of Romano's students using Romano's procedure, also introduced the idea of using a grooved director that was passed into the urethra and then cut down upon.

The "Marian operation" led the surgeon directly into the bladder and minimized accidental damage to neighboring tissues. Sounds, dilators, and forceps were used in addition to the knife; this gave it the name "the greater operation." The prostatic urethra was entered and dilated or torn through the perineal urethrotomy. It was treated like the female urethra once opened perineally; the stone, when grasped, was forcefully pulled out notwithstanding obstructions. The Italian surgeons showed the way in these new forms of lithotomy.

The descriptions of these operations always were very specific regarding positioning of the patient and holding him

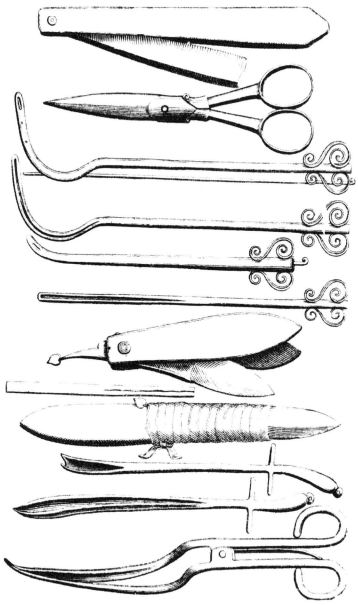

FIG. 2. *Lithotomy instruments. (From Tolet F: Traite de la Lithotomie. 4th Ed, Paris, 1689.)*

secured while the operation was accomplished. To get a better idea of some of these procedures, let us set the stage for the operation. First, let us look at the description in the *Sushruta Samhita,* the date estimated at 600 BC to 600 AD: When should an operation be done: *

A physician should have recourse to the following measures [surgery] in cases where the above-mentioned decoctions, medicated milk, alkalies, clarified butter, and littara-vasti [urethral syringe] of the aforesaid drugs would prove ineffective. Surgical operations in these cases do not prove successful, even in the hands of a skillful and experienced surgeon; so a surgical [lithotomic] operation should be considered a remedy that has little to recommend itself. The death of the patient is almost certain without a surgical operation, and the result to be derived from it is also uncertain. Hence, a skilled surgeon should perform such operations only with the permission of the king.

Preoperative preparations must include:

The patient should be soothed by the application of oleaginous substances, his system should be cleansed with emetics and purgatives and be slightly reduced thereby; he should then be formulated after being annointed with oily unguents, and be made to partake of a meal.

Prayers, offerings and prophylactic charms should be offered and the instruments and surgical accessories required in the case should be arranged in the order laid down.

It was very important that "the surgeon should use his best endeavours to encourage the patient and infuse hope and confidence in the patient's mind."

Operative preparation and positioning were detailed:

A person of strong physique and unagitated mind should be first made to sit on a level board or table as high as the knee joint. The patient should be made to lie on his back on the tables, placing the

* Bhishagratna KL: *An English Translation of the Sushruta Samhita.* Varanasi, Chowkhamba Sanskrit Series Office, 1963.

upper part of his body in the attendant's lap, with his waist resting on an elevated cloth cushion. Then the elbows and knee-joints (of the patient) should be contracted and bound up with fastenings or with linen (Fig. 3). After that the umbilical region (abdomen) of the patient should be well-rubbed with oil or with clarified butter and the left side of the umbilical region should be pressed down with a closed fist so that the stone comes within the reach of the operator.

The description of the operation is simplicity itself:

The surgeon should then introduce into the rectum the second and third fingers of his left hand, duly annointed and with the nails well pared. Then the fingers should be carried upwards toward the "rope" of the perineum in the middle line so as to bring the stone between the rectum and the penis, when it should be so firmly and strongly pressed as to look like an elevated tumour, taking care that the bladder remains contracted but at the same time even.

Even at this late point in preparations, the surgeon is warned that it's not too late to cancel:

An operation should not be proceeded with nor an attempt made to extract the stone in a case where, the stone on being handled, the patient would be found to drop down motionless [faint] with his head bent down and eyes fixed in a vacant stare like that of a dead man, as an extraction in such a case is sure to be followed by death. The operation should only be continued in the absence of such an occurrence.

The actual surgery was clearly described:

An incision should then be made on the left side of the raphe of the perineum at the distance of a barley corn and of a sufficient width to allow the free egress of the stone. Several authorities recommend the opening to be on the right side of the raphe of the perineum for the convenience of the operation. Special care should be taken in extracting the stone from its cavity so that it may not break into pieces nor leave any broken particles behind, however small, as they would,

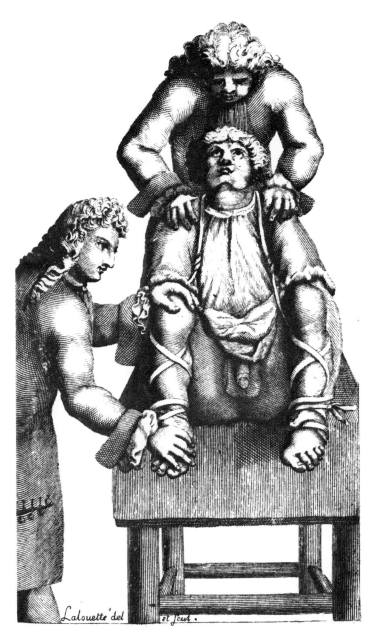

FIG. 3. *Lithotomy position. Note patient's expression. (From Tolet F: Trait de la Lithotomie. 4th Ed, Paris, 1689.)*

in such a case, be sure to grow larger again. Hence, the entire stone should be extracted.

Postop orders included:

After the extraction of a stone the patient should be made to sit in a Droni [cauldron] full of warm water and be fomented thereby. In doing so the possibility of an accumulation of blood in the bladder will be prevented; however if blood be accumulated therein, a decoction of the Kshira-trees should be injected into the bladder with the help of a urethral syringe.

These passages from the *Sushruta Samhita* should build an image of some of the earliest of these operations, but not those carried out in France in the 1500s. These surgical procedures were attended by both royalty and high society. If a wealthy patient had a stone, he would arrange to attend several sessions of surgery by various lithotomists and pick the one in whom he had the most faith. Popular lithotomists had sessions with limited paid admissions, and timing the surgery was a favorite pastime of the onlookers. The surgeon—in his velvet trousers, long flowing coat, and cap (Fig. 4) —was actor in and producer of the stone drama!

The story of Frère Jacques (1651–1714) is somewhat atypical, but still gives the flavor of the era.* He was first a cavalryman for five years; upon leaving the army he became a servant, or follower, of an Italian lithotomist. From him, Frère Jacques learned surgical technique and apparently became a very rapid and facile surgeon. He adopted the clothing and manners of the Monks, calling himself Frère Jacques. He was an itinerant lithologist, setting up operating clinics in the villages. Here he would line up his patients and prepare them for several days with clysters, bloodletting, and purges. On the day of surgery, he and four assistants operated on all his patients and then moved on before the results of the surgery

---

* Riches E: The history of lithotomy and lithotrity. *Ann Roy Coll Surg Eng 43:* 185–199, 1968.

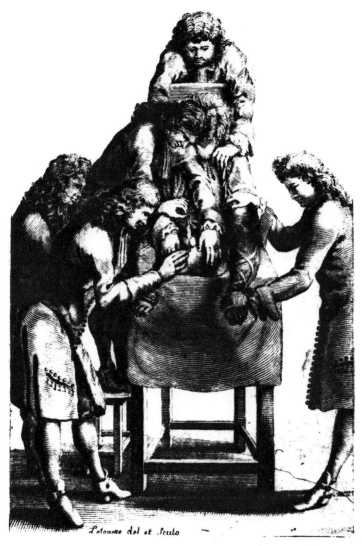

FIG. 4. *Lithotomy surgery. Note the surgical gowns. (From Tolet F: Traite de la Lithotomie. 4th Ed, Paris, 1689.)*

became known. Patients that died or developed fistulae or other complications were hardly good advertisements. The less skilled lithotomists preferred not to have many onlookers to witness the accidents. Frère Jacques permitted all to come. Although completely untaught in anatomy, he was proud of his manual dexterity. He boasted of his new methods of "cutting for stone," and went to Paris to teach the surgeons his procedures.

His new development in "cutting for stone" was the lateral approach to stone through the bladder. He used a solid grooveless metal staff which he passed into the bladder. He then incised the perineum two fingers medial to the tuberi ischii, carrying it forward from the anus. The bladder was thus opened and spread widely, and the stone was removed by forceps or fingers. This operation was much more satisfactory in adults than the midline or Celsurian approach. It permitted better access to the bladder while producing much less trauma to tissues. The midline approach was safely used in young children and youths, but in adults it was dangerous.

Frère Jacques applied for licensure or operating privileges at the Hôtel–Dieu and at the Charité Hospital in Paris, but was told he must first demonstrate on a cadaver that was then to be examined. He flunked this examination, although the surgeon was impressed with the facility of his surgery. He then went to Fontainebleau, where the Court physicians permitted him to operate on a lad. This boy lived and went home in three weeks. Frère Jacques was then held under the wing and in the favor of the king, and so was able to return later to Paris and successfully apply for privileges to practice there. He was finally in the position for which he had struggled; unfortunately, his errors caught up with him rapidly. He operated before crowds of up to 200 people. He "cut" sixty patients in a four-month period. Twenty-five died soon after surgery and thirteen were cured. The remaining twenty-two were beyond cure. On one day seven patients died; Frère Jacques accused the monks of Paris' famous Charité Hospital of poisoning his patients. Autopsies were performed and it was discovered that bladders were cut through, urethras severed and wounded in many places, with rectums and vaginas cut into as well! He then went back to his itinerant practice, setting out advertisements of his operation which "never endangered life."

He taught his "lateral operation" to many; when taught some anatomy himself, he modified his operation, using a grooved staff and a more anatomic approach. He also divided the prostate and bladder neck on the grooved director. He was then able to operate on thirty-eight patients without a death. He traveled from metropolis to metropolis, operating for the stone; he was given golden sounds and gold medals in recognition of his skills. He was said to have operated on 5000 patients. Royalty or high officials would often come to him desiring surgery for vesical calculi; they would observe him, and then hopefully submit to his knife. A traveling lithotomy table was often an essential piece of his equipment (Fig. 5).

After Frère Jacques, lithotomy leadership passed to William Cheselden (1688–1752) of England. Cheselden was a well-trained anatomist. He learned anatomy well, and he made careful anatomic dissection of cadavers before performing his surgery. He was a member of the Barber Surgeons Company and was probably one of the earliest teachers of anatomy in London. His *The Anatomy of the Human Body*, written when he was twenty-five, survived thirteen editions. Cheselden was also one of the earliest of English surgeons to use the "high operation," or suprapubic approach. He realized that the distended bladder carried the peritoneum upward with it and that an extraperitoneal approach was feasible. This operation he soon gave up, however, in favor of the perineal approach which was the style at that time.

John Douglas had introduced the suprapubic approach into England, and Cheselden adapted it for his own use. Cheselden found, however, that an unanesthetized patient's struggles and straining made a suprapubic operation dangerous, but actually aided the perineal approach by pushing bladder contents downward. He soon lost his enthusiasm for the procedure and went back to the perineal approach. This he modified into his

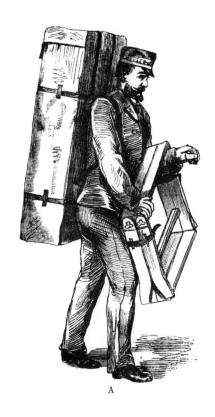

A

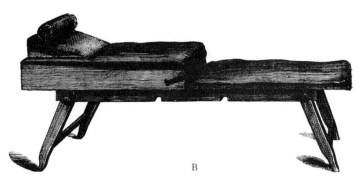

B

FIG. 5. *Ultzmann's portable lithotomy table. A. Traveling B. Ready for work (From Ultzmann Robert: Die Krankheiten der Harnblase. Stuttgart, Enke, 1890.)*

own procedure, which was then adopted by most of the Barber Surgeon lithotomists.

His technique he described as follows: *

I tie the patient as for the 'greater apparatus', but lay him upon a blanket several doubles upon an horizontal table three feet high, with his head only raised. I first make as long an incision as I can, beginning near the place where the old operation ends, cutting down between the musculus accelerator urinae, and erector penis, and by the side of the intestinum rectum: I then feel for the staff, holding down the gut all the while with one or two fingers of my left hand, and cut upon it in that part of the urethra which lies beyond the corpora cavernosa urethrae, and in the prostate gland, cutting from below upwards, to avoid wounding the gut; and then passing the gorget very carefully in the groove of the staff into the bladder, bear the point of the gorget hard against the staff, observing all the while that they do not separate, and let the gorget slip to the outside of the bladder; then I pass the forceps into the right side of the bladder, the wound being on the left side of the perinaeum; and as they pass, carefully attend to their entering the bladder, which is known by their overcoming a straitness which there will be in the place of the wound; then taking care to push them no farthur, so that the bladder may not be hurt. I first feel for the stone with the end of them, which having felt, I open the forceps and slide one blade underneath it, and the other at the top; and if I apprehend the stone is not in the right place in the forceps, I shift it before I offer to extract, and then extract it very deliberately, so that it may not slip suddenly out of the forceps, and that the parts of the wound may have time to stretch, taking great care not to gripe it so hard as to break it, and if I find the stone very large, I again cut upon it as it is held in the forceps. Here I must take notice, it is very convenient to have the bladder empty of urine before the operation, for if there is any quantity to flow out of the bladder at the passing in of the gorget, the bladder does not contract but collapses into folds, which makes it difficult to lay hold of the stone without hurting the bladder; but if the bladder is contracted, it is so easy to lay hold of it, that I have never been delayed one moment, unless the stone was

* Cheselden William: *The Anatomy of the Human Body.* 2nd Am ed Boston, David West, 1806.

very small. Lastly, I tie the blood vessels with the help of a crooked needle, and use no other dressing than a little bit of lint besmeared with blood, that it may not stick too long in the wound, and all the dressing during the cure are very slight, almost superficial, and without any bandage to retain them; because that will be wetted with urine, and gall the skin. At first I keep the patient very cool to prevent bleeding, and sometimes apply a rag, dipt in cold water, to the wound, and to the genital parts, which I have found very useful in hot weather particularly. In children it is often alone sufficient to stop the bleeding and always helpful in men. The day before the operation, I give a purge to empty the guts, and never neglect to give some laxative medicine or clyster a few days after, if the belly is at all tense, or if they have not a natural stool.

It is appropriate to conclude this chapter on lithotomy with a musical poem. Marin Marais, musician and composer of the era, underwent a lithotomy about 1715. As a result, he wrote the famous musical piece *Picture of an Operation for Stone*. The words to the music are:

> Appearance of the operating set up
> The patient shudders upon seeing it
> He resolves nevertheless to proceed.
> He climbs up and lies on the table
> His thoughts are somber
> Silken ties bind his arms to his hips.
> The incision is made.
> The grasping forceps is introduced.
> The stone is extracted.
> The patient is unable even to cry out.
> There is a rush of blood
> The ties are removed.
> The patient is taken to his bed.

Catheters

Emptying the painfully overfilled and unhappily obstructed bladder must have been one of the problems of man since Genesis. Urinary retention is mentioned in most of the earliest recorded histories. Catheterizations were reported to have been accomplished with reeds, straws, and curled-up palm leaves; the Chinese used "leaves of the allium" as well. This is too often quoted and then dropped. *Allium* is the generic name of the onion family and the long, thin leaves are hollow; if properly dried and prepared, they would make excellent catheters. In Figure 6, green bunching onions, also known as scallions, are photographed with a red rubber catheter to demonstrate their similarities. Breakage and the difficulty of pushing these treated leaves past obstructions soon resulted in improved instrumentation. Instead of the reed or the onion leaf, copper, bronze, and tin catheters were soon developed. The Sumerians, probably the antecedents of both the Babylonians and the Egyptians, may have even used gold to make catheters. Because it is soft and malleable, gold was ideally suited for this purpose. In the Vedas, some catheters were described as coated with lac and lubricated with ghee (from butter) .

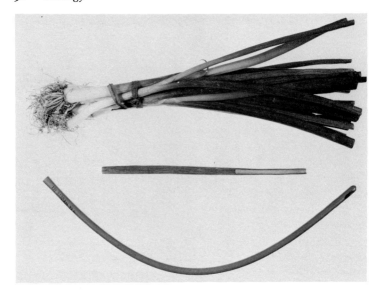

FIG. 6. *Bunching onions, red rubber catheter* (22 F), *and in the middle an allium leaf prepared as a catheter.*

In the excavations of Pompeii, catheters of metal were recovered; only shortly after that period, Galen (131–210 AD) demonstrated his now famous S-shaped metal catheter for use in both men and women. Indeed, as is often true with medical discoveries, Galen seems to have been antedated several hundred years by Erasistratos (circa 310–250 BC) of Keos, who is said to have used an S-shaped catheter he invented to treat strictures and urinary retention.

The next significant forward step is noted in Avicenna's description in 1036 of a flexible, or more likely malleable, catheter. Arculanis (who died about 1484) also mentioned flexible catheters. The silver catheter soon became the most popular. Silver was chosen for several reasons: It was easily formed, easily bent as desired, and was said to have some antiseptic function.

Then the woven catheter was produced and indeed, the silk

woven, varnished catheter is its direct descendant. The woven catheters were of tubular construction, soaked in linseed oil, and then dried. The silk woven coated catheter is of course much smoother, more regular, and more readily produced. It is also very hard to sterilize satisfactorily, and when old, very likely to break while in use, causing trauma and also some desperate searches for the lost intraurethral or intravesical portions. Louis Mercier (1811–1882) used the woven catheters first popularized by the German Johann Theden, and added curves and olivary bulges to form the identical shapes still in most frequent use today, known as the coudé and olive coudé. Coudé means elbow in French and indeed the catheters have an elbow-like bend near the distal end. The French terminology is still used because the French were then the foremost manufacturers of catheters, and the names stuck. They rapidly adopted rubber (or caoutchouc) and produced flexible catheters.

Benjamin Franklin, in 1752, described to his brother a silver catheter made so that it might be flexible, but must be covered with a "fine gut" or rubbed with tallow to fill the joints. Needless to say, the rubber ones were much more readily received and widely acclaimed.

Rubber could not be formed and shaped as desired until around 1844 when Goodyear hit on what is now known as vulcanization. In a short ten years, Auguste Nélaton of Paris had seen the value of this new process, and the Goodyear methods were used to produce what is still known and used as the Nélaton type of catheter: red rubber, solid tip, and one-eyed.

One of the oft-requested developments was a catheter that could be retained in place through its own configuration. Most indwelling catheters were taped or tied to the penis in men, and they were sometimes sewed to the urethral orifice in women. This was, of course, unsatisfactory in both cases.

In 1822, Theodore Ducamp used inflatable bags on his dilating bougies. The bags were formed of goldbeater's skin, a submucosal layer of the intestines of oxen, and were tied on catheters and inflated through the main lumen to distend the strictures. Reybard used this idea but soon developed it further and utilized a separate lumen to inflate the bag and maintain the catheter's normal functon. Thus, the first indwelling catheter was maintained in the bladder by the inflated bag, the Foley catheter's grandfather (Fig. 7).

Other ways to keep the catheter in the bladder were also demonstrated. In 1892, Dr. Malecot showed his four-winged catheter, followed shortly by the de Pezzer "mushroom" and others.

Ureteral catheters became important following the development of the cystoscope. When Gustav Simon first passed a catheter into the ureter on his finger tip, it was not a ureteral catheter, but a hollow probe. Now new, soft, fine, flexible catheters were needed. At first they were made without graduation marks and were not opaque to x-rays. The first production models manufactured by the great French company, Eynard, were probably designed by Dr. Joaquin Albarran, a renowned urologist who had originated many important urologic instruments, including the cystoscope's Albarran elevator. When roentgenography was made an integral part of the urologic workup, catheters opaque to x-rays were soon forthcoming. X-ray opaque ureteral catheters were rigged with inflatable balloons used to dilate strictures, and as described by R. L. Dourmashkin, to help deliver calculi.

The Foley catheter was the next big development in catheters. It was the offspring of many earlier attempts. Some of the more recent attempts are still slightly obscured by what may be called the lack of historic perspectives.

In 1955, Edson L. Outwin wrote:*

In 1927, there occurred what is probably the most epochal event affecting the development of the modern catheter. In April of that year, Dr. Theodore M. Davis of Greenville, South Carolina, resurrected the resectoscope invented by Dr. Maximilian Stern of New

* Outwin EL: The development of the modern catheter. *Amer Surg Trade Assoc J,* June, 1955.

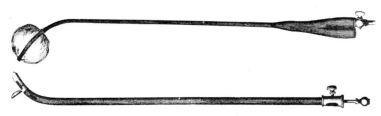

FIG. 7. *Early self-retaining catheters. (From Pousson A, Desnos E (eds) : Encyclopédie française d'Urologie. Paris, Doin et Fils, 1914–1923.)*

York City. Dr. Stern used his instrument during the early 20s on 46 cases which he reported on in 1927. However, other urologists could not obtain satisfactory results from his instrument because of their inability to control hemorrhage. While in New York waiting for the Wappler Electric Company, distributors of the Stern instrument, to locate one for him, Dr. Davis visited the Bard office and suggested to the writer that the hemorrhage resulting from cutting with the Stern technique might be controlled by attaching a balloon to a urethral catheter which, when inflated, would press against the severed blood vessels and act as a tourniquet until natural coagulation took place. The original drawing for this suggested balloon catheter is still in existence. However, this catheter never got beyond the drawing stage, as Dr. Davis, an expert with electrical devices, was able to improve both the resectoscope and the surgical diathermy unit with which it was used so that he could control hemorrhage by using two different currents, one for cutting and the other for coagulating. He, therefore, had no need for the balloon catheter in his practice. (In passing, credit should be given to Dr. Vincent J. Oddo of Providence, Rhode Island, for whom the writer in 1927 made a 5 cc balloon self-retaining catheter by tying a balloon made of prophylactic rubber to a two-way woven catheter.)

In use, this catheter proved impractical as the quality of rubber available at that time caused the balloon to disintegrate very soon after coming into contact with the urine in the bladder. It was not until latex rubber became available in the early 30s that the 5 cc balloon self-retaining catheter became practical.

The idea, however, was not restricted to Davis, for in 1930 Dr. F. E. B. Foley of St. Paul, Minnesota, had Bard import for him a longitudinally–grooved catheter to which he attached an inflating tube and a balloon by means of fine silk thread and waterproof cement. These catheters were ordered in 1929. During this period, Dr. Thomas M. Jarmon of Tyler, Texas, by a very ingenious method of tying on the bags, contributed considerably to the use of balloon catheters. About the same time, Dr. James W. Gerow of Reno, Nevada, was granted a patent for a balloon catheter which, as far as the records show, was never manufactured commercially. During this same period, Dr. Edgar G. Ballenger of Atlanta, Georgia, had Bard make for him a metal catheter with a rubber balloon tied on.

The first balloon catheter commercially manufactured and sold was presented to the profession by Dr. Hobart Dean Belknap of Portland, Oregon, in an article published in the 1933 issue of *The Urologic and Cutaneous Review*. This catheter was manufactured by a mechanical rubber molder in Portland and distributed by Bard. It was also during this period, in which the first catheters were made of which balloons were an integral part, that the Anode Company, with the help of Dr. Foley, produced a practical balloon catheter now known as the "Foley."

Following the development of the methods of molding red rubber and latex, plastics soon came of age, and both ureteral and urethral catheters were made of plastics of all colors and many consistencies. The goal of plastic makers and catheter manufacturers is to obtain a catheter that is soft yet firm, with a large lumen and small caliber, but with walls that won't collapse with suction, that will cause no tissue reaction, is indeed antibacterial, and yet will not give a foothold to concretions or crystals.

We have not as yet reached this desideratum.

Bladder Stones

Many were the ingenious ways attempted to diagnose and remove stones (Fig. 8). One gentleman used a curved sound with a roughened inside curve to saw away at his calculus. He passed the instrument into his bladder daily and worked on his stone to break it into small pieces that he passed readily. One fashioned a hollow sound and passed through it a small flexible file with which to cut upon his stone. Another ingenious device was the leather bag on a hollow handle (Fig. 9); this was collapsed and passed into the bladder. The stone was to be caught in the bag; the bag then closed and filled through the handle with acid. When the stone was dissolved, it was removed from the bag in the acid through the handle. The bag, collapsed again, could be removed from the bladder. Other instruments were fashioned with which to grasp stones and drill them or break them. Sanctorius fashioned an instrument with three arms, held together while being passed by a cap or a stem, so that it could be released inside the bladder (Fig. 10). Pulling back on the stylet permitted urine to drain and the arms to spread widely; then the smaller stones were pushed between the arms and the instrument was withdrawn through the urethra. Imagine the trauma of a larger stone

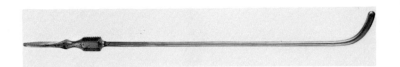

FIG. 8. *Stone "sounder" or "searcher." Passed into the bladder and twisted. If the flat sides hit a calculus a definite click was produced. (Courtesy of the Urology Museum, The Albert Einstein College of Medicine, New York City.)*

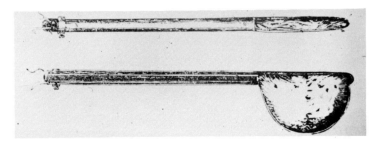

FIG. 9. *Bag for dissolution of stone. First, the tightly closed leather bag is passed into the bladder. It is opened and uncovered in the bladder and the stone is captured in the bag. The bag is then closed and filled with acid introduced through the handle. When the stone is dissolved, it is evacuated through the handle, and the bag is closed up and removed. This device probably was never used. (From Pousson A, Desnos E (eds): Encyclopédie française d'urologie. Paris, Doin et Fils, 1914–1923.)*

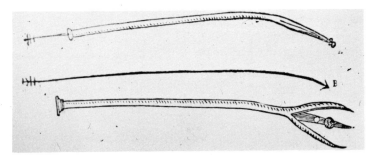

FIG. 10. *Sanctorius' stone forceps. It is passed with stylet in place. With stylet removed in the bladder, the arms are pressed open and urine is passed out through the stem. It was hoped that the stone would be held between the three blades as the instrument was removed. Obviously, only small stones were amenable. (From Pousson A, Desnos E (eds): Encyclopédie française d'urologie. Paris, Doin et Fils, 1914–1923.)*

lodged in the arms of this instrument! Sanctorius invented this particular instrument for a stone that he himself had.

Many were the adaptations of this type of forceps. The hollow stem was used to carry sharp penetrating points, drills, hammers, and even chemicals. Some used acids in the bladder; lime was also used in attempting to reduce the size of, and pain from, the stone.

Fournier de Lempdes (1783–1848) invented an instrument he named the Litholepte. This ingeniously manufactured machine was passed as a straight rod. Once inside the water-filled bladder it could be enlarged to form a cage in which to catch the stone and break it into small pieces eventually to be passed per urethrum. This was demonstrated on a cadavar, but it may never have been used on a living patient.

The French were supreme in manipulations and extractions of stones. They invented instruments to crush stones, to break them up, to drill them, and then to catch and remove the stones. Jean Civiale's trilabe was the first of many new French instruments (Fig. 11).

Other instruments of about that time were made for the purpose of breaking up a stone. The stone was first to be caught in the blades of the instrument, and then reduced in size by drills—some of them diamond-tipped—which were turned (Fig. 12). A bow was used with some of these instruments in order to turn the drill fast enough to fracture the stone (Figs. 13 and 14). If the stone was large, its parts were caught and drilled again and again until small enough to be removed transurethrally. Other ways of breaking the stone were sought by Leroy d'Étiolles with his lithoprione, a sort of metal basket that could be brought together with some force. He also modified Civiale's trilabe by adding a sharp instrument in the center to break the calculus once it was grasped.

Leroy d'Étiolles was given many prizes and awards in honor of his work in this field. In 1825, a French Prize Commission gave an honorable mention "To M. Amussat for making known the structure of the urethra and so making it easier to pass and use lithotritic instruments, to M. Civiale for applying

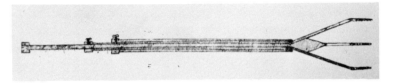

FIG. 11. Trilabe; Civiale's first model used to crush stones. (From Pousson A, Desnos E (eds): Encyclopédie française d'urologie. Paris, Doin et Fils, 1914–1923.)

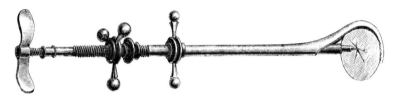

FIG. 12. Screw-type drill to catch and fragment stones. (From Ultzmann Robert: Die Krankheiten der Harnblase. Stuttgart, Enke, 1890.)

these instruments for the first time in humans, and to M. Leroy d'Étiolles for having thought of them, having them made, and having made known successively the refinements which he suggested for them." In 1826, the commission ". . . unanimously gave an award of two thousand francs to M. Leroy d'Étiolles, who published in 1825 a summary of lithotritic methodology and who was the first, in 1822, to make known these instruments which he had invented." In 1828, a further award and in 1831, six thousand francs "for a discovery, every day more appreciated . . . applications which he has made to lithotrite of the three-armed forceps, instrument most essential . . ." His work continued, and others developed other attacks on the stone (Fig. 15).

Several instruments of a similar type with points or rasps or files were devised, and Baron Herteloup first used the instrument from which the modern lithotrite was developed. His "percuteur" was to catch the calculus between two blades and then use a hammer or mallet externally to push the smaller

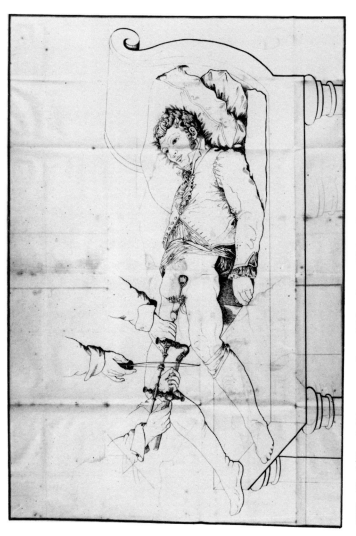

FIG. 13. *Lithontripteur a archet. Lithotrity utilizing bow lithotrite to drill and break stone. (From Dr. Civiale über die Lithotritie. Breslau, 1827).*

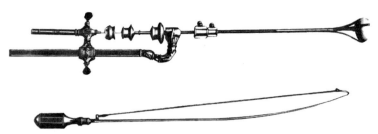

FIG. 14. *Lithotrite being used in Figure 13. (From Pousson A, Desnos E (eds): Encyclopédie française d'urologie. Paris, Doin et Fils, 1914–1923.)*

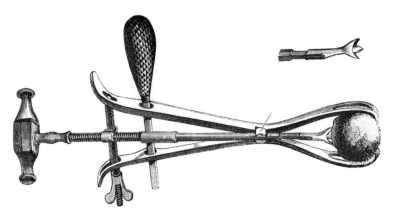

FIG. 15. *Screw lithotrite, two-bladed, for female patients. (From Ultzmann Robert: Die Krankheiten der Harnblase. Stuttgart, Enke, 1890.)*

blades against and into the large distal one (Fig. 16). Joseph Charrière probably used this instrument with the addition of rack and pinion or screw for pressure to break the stone without use of a hammer (Fig. 17).

Dr. Henry J. Bigelow, a Boston urologist, made a large advance towards safe lithotrity. In a book, *Rapid Lithotrity with Evacuation*, published in 1878, he first described his

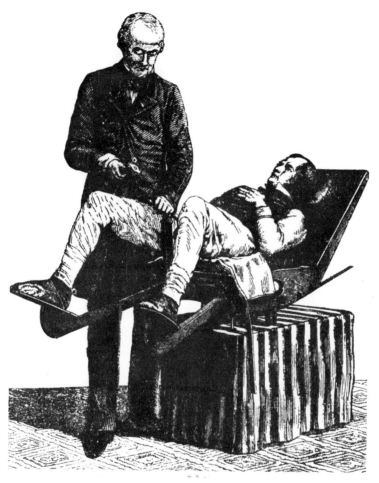

FIG. 16. *Herteloup's percussion stone breaker. A hammer was used to drive the drill into and through the stone. (From Pousson A, Desnos E (eds): Encyclopédie française d'urologie. Paris, Doin et Fils, 1914–1923.)*

methods: how to fill the bladder, crush the calculi, and wash out the particles. This operation, "litholapaxy," is still done the same way to this day. Younger urologists often stand in awe as the older man crushes a large stone with the "blind" lithotrite (Fig. 18). Without this maneuver, vesicolithotomy might have been needed as modern lithotrites with telescopes cannot grasp or crush the really large stones. The mortality from stone crushing dropped tremendously once this type of procedure became known and used.

Bigelow modified the ends of the crushing instruments due to several weaknesses in the ones in use. Because of their shape, the instruments were traumatic to pass. Also, the grasping parts needed to interlock closely, presenting a smooth surface for manipulation. The blades, therefore, were often so weak they broke very easily. Bigelow used fenestrae for better mating of the halves, and so increased their strength as well. He then experimented with vacuum bottles to withdraw fluid and particles and to wash out fragments. These proved to be too cumbersome, so he tried rubber bulbs for suction and appended small glass bottles in order to see and collect the pieces. These have now been modified into the evacuators that are seen in most cystoscopy suites today. They are now used more often for transurethral resections than for litholapaxies.

Many were the attempts with caustics, acids, and other chemicals to dissolve vesical calculi. The highest hopes were that a medication might be discovered that, when taken by mouth, would cause dissolution of the stone already formed in the bladder without causing damage to other organs or systems.

In 1739, Theophilus Lobb, M.D., published *Treatise on Dissolvents of the Stone; and on Curing the Stone and Gout by Aliment*. This work, with experiments, cases, and observations, was in its greatest part previously presented to the Royal Society of London, and it was printed as a result of the desire of the members of the Society. In his book Lobb states that animal foods and the neglect of exercise are the principal causes of both stone and gout. He then describes all the ex-

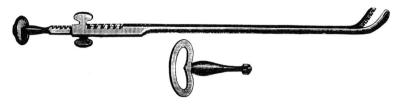

FIG. 17. *Charriere's lithotrite. This may have been the first rack-and-pinion lithotrite. (From Ultzmann Robert: Die Krankheiten der Harblase. Stuttgart, Enke, 1890.)*

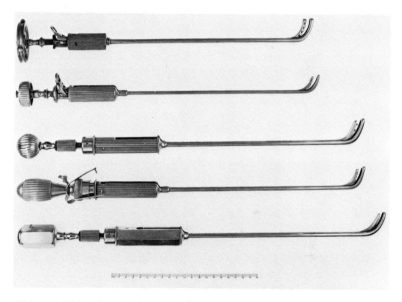

FIG. 18. *Lithotrites in the collection of the Urology Museum of the Albert Einstein College of Medicine, New York City.*

periments he used to dissolve stones *in vitro*. He used vinegar, pump water, cider, celery juice, grapes, currants, cucumber juice, cabbage juice, lemon juice, mulberry juice, onions, pears, raisins, tea, port wine, and brandy. Without knowledge of the composition of stones, he soaked them in various combinations of readily available materials to see if they would dissolve: "What I mean by the word dissolve, in the column of events, is such a Dissolution of the Cohesion of the parts of the Calculus, that it broke into a sand or very small parts by a gentle feeling it."

Later he further elucidates:

If I had a stone in my bladder, I should desire it might never be broken into fragments, nay I would shun, as poison, everything, whether aliment or medicine that was likely to break it: But I should wish to have it dissolved, that is the Cohesion of its parts gradually destroyed . . . so the disunited particles, exceedingly minute will be continuously washed off from the stone, by the flowing of the urine, and with it carried out of the body.

He concludes his book with a full chapter of dietary instructions for those suffering from stone, gout, or both. He is strong on vegetables, vegetable juices, and liquors—wines, beers, and fruit juices. He didn't prohibit meats, but advised increased fluid intake with them.

Joanna Stephens became well known at this time because of her secret medication to dissolve stones. She sold this medication at a good price, and because a large group of her patients claimed cures, she became wealthy. There was a public clamor for her formula so that poor as well as wealthy might be cured of this very prevalent and painful disease. She refused to reveal her secret until she was quite wealthy and then gracefully acceded to an offer of 5000 pounds made by Parliament in England. She then presented this famous mixture to the Royal Society of London on January 14, 1741. In 1742, John Rutty, M.D., published a book entitled *Account of Some New Experiments and Observations on Joanna Stephens' Medicine* *for the Stone.* This gave the medication and "some hints for reducing it from an empirical to a rational use." The recipe as published in the *London Gazette* consisted of mixtures of egg-shells, snails, old clay pipes, swine's cresse, saxifrage, soap, burdock, seeds, haws and hips, and other commonly available materials. It has been reported that many of her certified cures were found to have stones remaining in their bladders after death. Before this, however, serious attention was given to it by the doctors and especially Rutty, who further goes on to state:*

The world has lately been favored with a new discovery of a remedy said to be effectual, and to be taken internally with safety. . . . The Instances of the Success with which the medicines have been used, deserve the serious Attention of Physicians, and ought to excite them to a careful examination of their effects, so as to render this discovery as useful to the public as the nature of this thing will admit, and as the British Parliament generously intended it to be.

The medicine was composed of many parts, "several parts of it being of little or no use, and others plainly calculated to disguise the rest." Several physicians examined the list of contents, and reduced the "pompous Medicine to a slacked'd Powder of calcined egg-shells, and a Solution of Soap. . . ."

According to Rutty, the doctors working to test this combination differentiated carefully between stone solvents and lithontriptics as follows:

. . . if by Solvent we understand that which effects such a comminution of the Parts of the Stone, as keeps them suspended in the Pores of the Menstruum, I know of nothing which lays claim to that title but Spirit of Nitre; the several Ingredients of this Medicine, which are to be the subject of the following Series of Experiments, do only corrode and precipitate the Parts of the Stones, and therefore in

* Rutty John: *Account of Some New Experiments and Observations on Joanna Stephens' Medicine for the Stone,* London, printed for R Manby, 1742.

Strictness should seem rather to deserve the Appellation of "lithon-tripticks" than Solvents.

The doctors used various solutions of soaps and found that stones both hard and soft became friable and formed powders. They also found lime—calcined lime—did the same *in vitro*.

Theophilus Lobb, M.D., F.R.S., in 1739 had listed in his book (previously mentioned) vegetables, familiar in most kitchens, that were noted for their lithontriptic effect on stones *out of the body.* So Rutty while trying Joanna Stephens' medicament also tried in comparison three of Lobb's and found them less useful. Understand, all of these were used *in vitro.* The only *in vivo* results were from uncontrolled case reports. Dr. James Jurin, having found himself suffering from the stone and almost incapacitated—he could no longer ride in his carriage because of pain—decided to treat himself with lithontriptics. He believed that Joanna Stephens' concoction was too nauseating to take so he decided to try the lixivium, or lye, of which soap is made, notwithstanding its caustic effect. He started with small doses, and he increased the dosage to his tolerance and passed gravel, sand, particulate matter, and finally three stones. He was certain he had stopped forming more stones when he noted his urine no longer "furred the sides of the chamber pot." He started with twenty drops and worked up to 1 or 1½ ounces a day. So the lithontriptics were widely used and accepted in England and Europe. Because so many suffered from this widely known and feared disorder, the many therapies attempted were not surprising.

Renal Surgery

Stones have been discussed to this extent because at present there is nothing resembling the number of stones of those early years. Pediatricians today do not think that a crying child may be suffering from vesical calculi. Doctors then considered it to be one of the most frequent causes of pain in children. We do not understand why there are not as many cases of stones now as then; but they certainly were very common. Not only vesical calculi, but also renal calculi were frequently seen.

The primary cause is still far from understood, but the frequency of stones in Europe in the last century has been called endemic.We have often tried to link urolithogenesis to nutrition and this certainly may have been one of the causes of stone in Europe in the eighteenth and nineteenth centuries. The marked increase in frequency of stones after the World Wars also could be based on nutritional factors. The high rates of stone in India, Japan, the Near East, and other areas even now may well be due to nutritional defects. Vesical calculi outnumber renal calculi, and most of the stones are of uric acid or ammonium and acid urates. Children are more often affected in these areas than adults. Today in Thailand a

situation similar to that in Europe in the eighteenth and nineteenth centuries seems to exist. But now, as then, we are still
not sure of the etiology. Then, as now, medical men, witch
doctors, and savants of all descriptions had their favorite
methods for treating stones.

Surgery for renal stone was prohibited by Hippocrates who
thought it too dangerous. He suggested that only nephric
abscesses be opened. Of course, most untended, uncared for
infected stones produce ruptures of the kidney and perinephric abscesses. So, opening perinephric abscesses produced some
stones, but doctors for the most part heeded Hippocrates'
warning and refused to operate for kidney stone.

Until the time of Vesalius (1514–1564), there was little
understanding of renal physiology nor had the anatomy been
studied because of restrictions against examining the human
body. It was common belief that the kidney consisted of two
chambers separated by a filter (Fig. 19). The blood came to
the upper chamber via the artery, circulated there while the
"noxious poisons" were filtered out as urine into the lower
chamber. The blood, filtered of its poisons, then left via the
exiting vein. The urine in the lower chamber was funneled
into the ureter and flowed gently to the bladder. The studies
of Vesalius proved the falsity of this conception, but the filtra-
tion theory prevailed for years after the complete anatomy was
known.

About 1680, Domenic deMarchetti, M.D., opened up the
entire field of kidney surgery. A Mr. Hobson, then the English
Consul in Venice, had renal colic. It was so severe and unre-
mitting that he was unable to work or to enjoy life. He
searched for some relief and went to doctor after doctor for
help. Finally, he went to deMarchetti and demanded that this
fine surgeon operate on his kidney. The request was refused.

The Consul then said, as patients to this day still say: "If
you won't do the surgery, I'll keep looking until I find a
surgeon who will, and I'd rather have you do it, as you're the
best." deMarchetti gave in. He studied what little was known of
spear and arrow wounds and then commenced to operate on

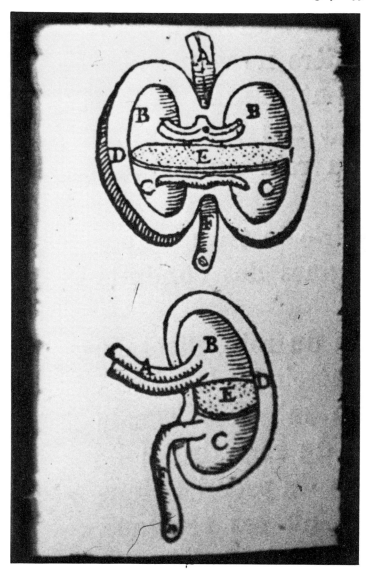

FIG. 19. *The anatomy of the kidney, as theorized before Vesalius. (From Pousson A, Desnos E (eds): Encyclopédie française d'urologie. Paris, Doin et Fils, 1914–1923.)*

Hobson's loin. This was still before anesthesia and prior to any knowledge of hemostasis. deMarchetti cut down to the kidney, but then there was such profuse bleeding that he packed the incision and sent the patient to bed. Next day the patient persuaded the surgeon to continue; he removed the packing and boldly incised the bulging kidney. There was a gush of purulent matter and urine, and half a dozen stones were delivered into the wound. The patient was immediately freed of his pain, and colic occurred no more. He had a persistent draining urinary fistula for several years until the remaining obstructing stone was vomited from the kidney and the wound healed.

Little further was done to advance renal surgery until near the turn of the century when Étienne Blancard did some experimental work in dog surgery. He proved—to his satisfaction at any rate—that dogs could live after the extirpation of one healthy kidney. It had long been known that animals survived when sick or wounded kidneys were removed accidentally or by mistake, but no one knew how an animal would fare if a healthy kidney were suddenly extirpated. Blancard proved that one healthy kidney was enough. He suggested to his medical confreres that in cases of persistent renal colic, nephrectomy would be valuable and cure the patient. His colleagues listened and laughed, and there was no further renal surgery for years.

About 1756, Prudent Hévin was commissioned by the Royal Academy of Surgery in Paris to study the possibility of "nephrectomy surgery". He investigated past studies and recent work, and concluded that the only safe surgery was drainage of renal abscesses and not nephrectomy.

Hévin pushed renal surgery back another hundred years, in much the same manner as had Galen years before. The latter had negated Hippocrates' work very easily. Hippocrates had drained tuberculous and nontuberculous pyonephrosis, as well as pyelonephritic abscess, and had incised swellings of the loin due to stone. Celsus revived these almost forgotten works of the master in his book *De Re Medica,* but not being a doctor he apparently confused renal and bladder stones. Celsus thought all renal wounds to be fatal and this, when published in his great book of medical knowledge, stopped renal surgery. Galen, another hundred years later, wrote about lithiasis extensively. He described clots in the bladders of patients with wounded kidneys, but he too believed that surgical intervention was fatal.

Aetius, the Mesopotamian, pointed out that persistent fistulae often followed the drainage of renal abscesses secondary to stone and tuberculosis. Kidney surgery was usually fatal. Thus, some 700 years later, Hippocrates' observations were again advanced. Still no surgeons dared elective renal surgery. Still later, in the eleventh century, some little-known Arab physician advised operating on the kidney for stone. It was not considered ethical, however, and we don't know if it was attempted.

The famous case of the condemned archer Bagnolete is in many of our medical history books, but little is known except that this man was said to have had a renal calculus. To escape the hangman, he agreed to allow surgery on his kidney on the condition that, if he survived, he would be freed. He survived and was freed in 1474. Still, renal surgery was considered too dangerous by ethical physicians.

Giuseppe Zambeccari, a pioneer in experimental surgery in 1670, Rounhyzer in 1672, and Étienne Blancard in 1690 performed their dog surgery, and each suggested that nephrectomy might be a therapeutic approach to renal lithiasis.

After Hévin's survey another hundred years passed before renal surgery again came to the fore. At that time Gustav Simon was doing surgery in Heidelberg, Germany. He was "Der Herr Professor," and difficult cases of all types were referred to him. Margaretha Kleb was one such difficult case. She had been operated on and a large ovarian cyst had been removed one-and-a-half years earlier. After this surgery, urine leaked from her abdomen and her vagina. To quote Simon: "The woman is always wet, she smells of rancid urine and nauseates her environment and herself." Simon's diagnosis was a masterpiece. He passed a probe through the abdominal fistula into the vagina through the cervix. This explained the purulent and bloody urine. Then he dilated the fistulous tract, found the ureteral orifice, and introduced a probe up to the left kidney. He satisfied himself that the bladder was intact by filling it with milk and not recovering any of that from the fistula or vagina. Simon tried five different times to close the fistula or stop the urine flow, but to no avail. "Now only extirpation of the kidney remains to be done." Put yourself, if you can, in Simon's position. Although there were articles describing three unintentional surgical extirpations of kidneys in humans, none of the patients had survived more than a few days, even though all three had "put out urine." Let's leave Ms. Kleb for the moment and examine the three cases.

It all began in 1809 when Ephraim McDowell performed the first successful elective abdominal surgery for removal of an ovarian cyst. Suddenly surgeons from all over began cutting for ovarian tumors. Ovariotomies—removal of the ovaries, usually for cysts—became quite commonplace. These were usually rough, gross operations, and done in the beginning without the aid of anesthesia. Speed was therefore essential, and so it isn't surprising that kidneys were removed accidentally as other abdominal lesions were excised.

Probably the first recorded nephrectomy was accomplished accidentally by Erastus Bradley Wolcott in 1861 when he operated to remove a cystic tumor of the liver. He didn't realize he had taken out the kidney until the specimen was cut for examination. His patient died in fifteen days from "exhaustion caused by infection." Otto Spiegelberg, in Germany, operated to remove an ovarian cyst; the specimen proved to be kidney infected with echinococcus. His patient died in 24 hours. The third patient was thought to have an ovarian tumor. Her kidney was removed transperitoneally by Edmund Peaslee; three days later she was dead, a victim of peritonitis.

Now Simon thought, from his experiments in animal surgery, that extirpation of a kidney was no more dangerous than hysterectomy. He knew a human could live with one kidney, but he didn't know if removal of a healthy kidney would leave enough functioning renal tissue behind to support life. He had no kidney function tests to help him, either. He wasn't even sure that he could ligate the renal artery, or if it would blow out when the sutures were removed. Finally, he wasn't sure he could do the operation retroperitoneally, and entering the peritoneum increased the risk tremendously. But Gustav Simon decided that it could be done, that the patient's suffering warranted the attempt, and that success meant cure.

He studied reports of animal surgery, of autopsies of patients with one kidney, and of the physiologists Claude Bernard and Pierre-François-Olive Rayer. Rayer, incidentally, found the procedure of value and safe in dogs, but too dangerous because of surgical technical difficulties to try in man. Simon operated on 30 dogs himself; he was aware of compensatory hypertrophy of the solitary kidney and was reassured that one kidney would produce a satisfactory physiologic result.

On August 2, 1869, in an amphitheater in Heidelberg before an illustrious audience of physicians, Simon explained the patient's situation and then removed the perfectly healthy, functioning kidney. With chloroform anesthesia, a lateral incision was made and the kidney exposed in ten minutes. The entire pedicle and ureter were mass ligated and the kidney amputated. The operation lasted forty minutes and the silk pedicle ligatures were led out of the incision. The patient's course was stormy. Her fever was elevated for seven weeks. She had a severe wound infection—"diphtheria and erysipelas" of the wound caused chills and fever. After six months the sutures were removed and the patient discharged. The picture of the obese Margaretha Kleb viewing her incision in front of a mirror is probably one of the best known medical illustrations. Simon's second planned nephrectomy was done on a woman from the United States. She died of sepsis when the surgeon found it necessary to probe the wound during her convalescence.

Nephrectomy didn't become common after Simon's cases, but several were done. A completely successful operation was performed on a woman five months pregnant in 1871. In contrast, a kidney with calculous pyonephrosis was removed from a patient who died shortly thereafter. Autopsy proved the opposite kidney had previously been destroyed by "abscess formation."

The limiting factor in many of these cases was the complete lack of knowledge of individual renal function and also a lack of diagnostic tests to determine the true condition of either kidney. Kidney disease often was not detected until it was so far advanced that unilateral nephrectomy was impossible. The cystoscope was not invented until 1878, and ureteral catheterization was not clinically used for another ten years. But this is another chapter in urologic history.

Renal Function Tests

As renal physiology advanced, it became more and more important to be able to tell how the individual kidneys functioned. In 1875, Gustav Simon digitally dilated the urethra of a woman and passed a catheter into the ureters on his finger (Fig. 20). This obviously gave him the urines from the separate kidneys, but it was not accomplished easily enough to be often repeated. Few had the intestinal fortitude to try.

Because of increasing knowledge of physiology and urinalysis and the importance of the kidneys, many were searching for methods of obtaining separate urines for examination. One instrumental technique of obtaining urines from each kidney separately was tried by Maro Tuchmann in London. He conceived the idea of compressing one ureteral orifice and obtaining urine from the other, then reversing the ureteral compressor and receiving urine from the second kidney. This instrument was a smooth-jawed, obliquely directed clamp that was capable of causing considerable damage.

Other instruments utilized rubber bags which, when overlying a ureteral orifice, were filled with mercury and were expected to halt urine output from that orifice. Rochet and Pellande invented another type of balloon obstructor attached

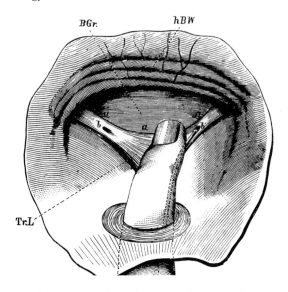

FIG. 20. *Using a finger through the urethra to catheterize a ureter, as described by Gustav Simon. (From Ultzmann Robert: Die Krankheiten der Harnblase. Enke, Stuttgart, 1890.)*

to a split hollow sound. One side was mobile; thus, one side could push the balloon against an orifice while the other side collected urine.

Polk and Eberman attempted to utilize pressure on the orifice against counterpressure in the rectum to compress the orifices. Nicolich probably came up with the simplest maneuver by simply collecting bladder urine while compressing one ureter by pressure on the anterior abdominal wall. He stated this test was only valuable when the differences in the urine were quite clear.

All these methods, it is easy to see, were complicated and some were dangerous. They couldn't be relied on in all cases and, usually when most needed, none would be suitable.

The thought that perhaps the bladder might be temporarily

divided into two reservoirs for the collection of urine—half for each kidney—was acted on separately by several men.

In 1891, Lambotte of Brussels invented an instrument useful only in women. This had two semicircular halves; each pressed down on one side of the bladder to make two drainage pools. Newman, a German, developed an instrument with a broad base and collecting parts at each extremity; when this was introduced into the bladder and a finger inserted vaginally to tent the floor, two pools were formed. This, of course, was of no use in men.

Luys invented an instrument with a rubber dam that was to divide the bladder into two halves. Part of the instrument was a catheter on each side of the dam. With the instrument in place and partitioning the bladder, urine from each kidney pooled on each side of the bladder and drained out the separate catheters (Fig. 21).

Harris made up another urine segregator (Fig. 22). One leaf of this instrument was placed in the vagina or rectum and tented the bladder floor in the midline, making two pools of urine, one from each side. A silver double catheter was passed into the bladder and opened widely apart, so that one catheter was in each pool of urine.

Luys' instrument failed in the face of any irregularity of the bladder wall such as tumor, diverticulum, and even trabeculation. Harris' instrument worked better unless there was a frozen pelvis or inflammatory changes in the floor of the bladder that prevented its elevation. Harris' instrument also was quite difficult to use in males of the prostatic age group. Other instruments were devised to separate the urine from each kidney so that chemical determination might reveal renal function. These were used often until the ureterocystoscope was invented, making it easier to collect urine directly from each renal pelvis for separate renal function studies.

Harris' instrument was actually used into the 1900s. At a large medical meeting in 1900, all these methods were discussed and ureteral catheterization was found to be the only

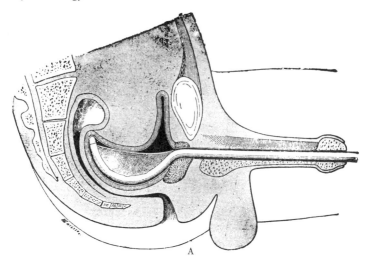

A

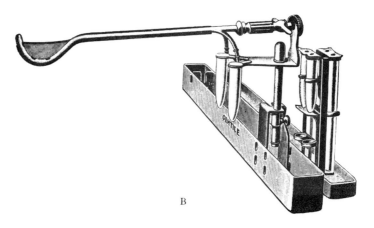

B

FIG. 21. *A. Luy's separator, used to divide a bladder into two segments to collect urines from each kidney. (From von Bergmann E, Von Bruns, P: A System of Practical Surgery. Philadelphia, Lea Bros, 1904) B. The instrument shown being used in part A. (Illustration supplied with instrument, courtesy of Urology Museum, The Albert Einstein College of Medicine, New York City.)*

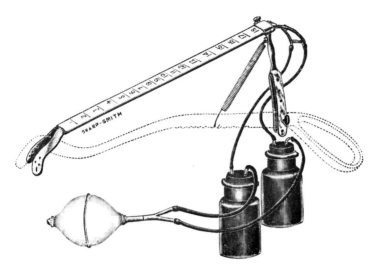

FIG. 22. *Harris' segregator. The lower piece tents up the floor of the the bladder and the two hollow halves of the main part spread out, one to each side, catching the urine flowing from each ureter. This was used to estimate individual renal function (From JAMA, 30: 236–238, Jan, 1898.)*

reliable way of obtaining separate urines for the study of individual renal function. Luys' instrument was probably used more often than any other instrument for this purpose before the popularization of ureteral catheterization. It worked fairly well in women and young men but poorly in older men.

Cathelin devised an instrument known as the "graduated divider of Cathelin." This combined the dividing membranes of Luys with the bifid mobile curved catheters of Harris, in one instrument. This was more reliable in men of all ages.

Boddaert invented a similar instrument, but his divider was a rubber cover over a mobile extension. Thus, the instrument could be opened to form a divider for the base of the bladder. It, too, was a combination of the Luys and Harris ideas.

But none of these were nearly as reliable as ureteral catheterization. Few were able or desirous of using Gustav Simon's digital methods, yet catheters must be placed in ureteral orifices. They badly needed further development of the cystoscope to make this a practical, safe, and easy measure available to all urologists.

Development of the
Cystoscope

For centuries man had sought the ability to search into the
cavity of the human body before death. Bivalved speculae and
other probes had given minimal entry, but until 1807 nothing
offered major advancement. Then Philipp Bozzini of Frank-
fort designed an instrument that was an elongated, very thin
funnel that could be passed into a large orifice. There was a
light carrier stand into which the proximal end of this funnel
could be fitted (Fig. 23A). In the stand was placed a candle;
the user's eye was protected from the candlelight by a reflector
which beamed candlelight down the funnel. Half the orifice
was for light and half for sight. Crude as it was, this was an
opening into the body and a way of lighting the tissues at the
distal end. Funnels of different sizes could be fitted and even a
bivalved funnel was adapted for use (Fig. 23B). The instrument was coarse, cumbersome, and even somewhat dangerous
to use because the candle heated its stand when it was held at
an angle. The Faculty of Medicine of Vienna, to whom
Bozzini presented his instrument, was less than overjoyed at
the invention. (There is no indication that it was ever used on

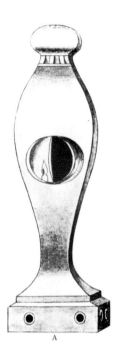

A

a human.) They complained it was too painful to introduce, the area illuminated was too small, and the illumination was insufficient. It was true, however, that most of the instruments that immediately followed the first Lichtleiter were derived from Bozzini's brainchild.

Pierre Ségalas presented his new instrument to the Academy of Sciences in 1826. This was a simplification of the Lichtleiter. It also was a funnel and was intended to illuminate the bladder and ureteral orifices. Ségalas named it the "urethrocystique speculum" (Fig. 24). The instrument was composed of silver tubes, the interiors of which were highly polished to reflect light. There was a hard rubber device to act as stylet and introducer. Two small candles and a concave mirror to focus the light formed the sole illumination, and an eyeshield gave protection to the operator from the candlelight. This instrument was used more easily, although the dangers of

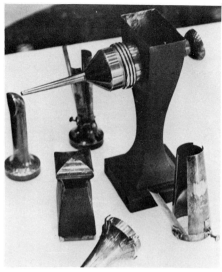

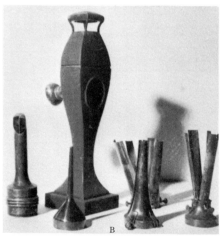

FIG. 23. *A. Bozzini's Lichtleiter, the first endoscope. Candlelight was used. (From Casper Leopold: Handbuch der Cystoskopie. Leipzig, 1911.) B. Two views of Philipp Bozinni's Lichtleiter. (Courtesy of the Museum of American College of Surgeons, Chicago.)*

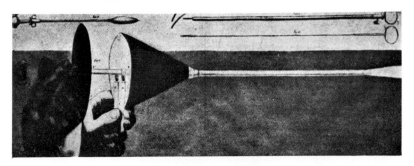

FIG. 24. *The Segalas endoscope, called the "speculum urethro-cystique." Two "candle power," with funnel and mirror. (From Pousson A, Desnos E, (eds): Encyclopédie française d'urologie. Paris, Doin et Fils, 1914–1923.)*

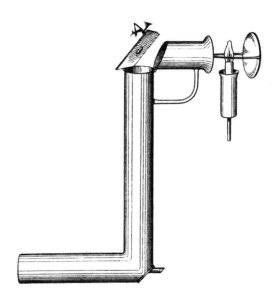

FIG. 25. *Fisher's cystoscope. (From Pousson A, Desnos E (eds): Encyclopédie française d'urologie. Paris, Doin et Fils, 1914–1923.)*

working between the legs with two lit candles cannot be "lightly" dismissed!

A Bostonian, Dr. John Fisher, published the invention of his cystoscope one year later, but stated he had developed his invention before Ségalas. The ensuing squabble was not decided to the satisfaction of Fisher. The date of publication is and was all-important in these arguments of priority. Fisher's cystoscope was amazingly unlike the Ségalas instrument in form, although both used the same principles. Fisher's instrument consisted of two right-angle turns of hollow tubing, forming a Z-like shape (Fig. 25). One end was introduced into the bladder; the other end carried the candle and concave mirror. The urologist, with the aid of mirrors, only looked around one corner, but the light was reflected around two. The image that reached the eye was reflected from the mirror and was reversed. Later on, this same instrument was fitted with an electric light by Professor Patterson. It was still not very satisfactory.

In 1853, Antonin Desormeaux presented to the Academy of Medicine an instrument based on a different principle (Fig. 26). His also was an elongated funnel, either straight or curved, that could be used in different sizes. But there the resemblance ends. Desormeaux's source of light was a wick burning alcohol that was held in a reservoir at the base of the handle. Here again the light was reflected into the organ by a concave mirror with a small central hole for the observer's eye. He was able to use instruments, and performed diagnostic tests and treatments of diseases of the ureters and even of ureterostomies. He reported vesical calculi seen with his endoscope, as well as ureteral mucoceles (or ureteroceles). He is often, and probably correctly, referred to as the "father of cystoscopy."

In 1865, Francis Richard Cruise demonstrated his modification of Desormeaux's instrument to the Medical Society of the King and Queen's College of Physicians (Figs. 27 and 28). His instrument was much like the original except the light source was placed to the side of the funnel and directed into it at

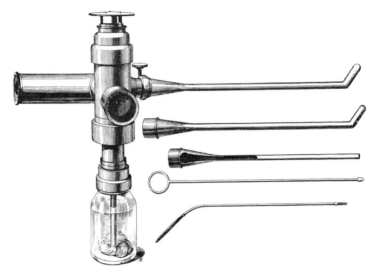

FIG. 26. *The Desormeaux alcohol lamp scope. (From Les Instruments de Chirurge Urinaire en France. Paris, Octave Pasteau, 1914.)*

right angles by a mirror. The light source itself is described by Cruise as follows:*

Experiments which I need not recall here, but which are familiar to those who have made investigations with polarized light, led me to the knowledge that one of the brightest illuminations which can be obtained by any means is that given off by the *thin edge of the flat flames* of the petroleum lamp. Moreover the steadiness and intensity of the light are increased to the utmost by using a tall draught chimney, and by dissolving camphor in the petroleum. . . .

Cruise admitted to two major faults with this instrument: it became very hot; and the light rays were so narrow that a very fine adjusting apparatus was required. He overcame the heat problem by making the lantern of mahogany so that it could

* Cruise FR: The endoscope as an aid in the diagnosis of disease. *Dublin Quart J Med Sci 39:* 329–363, No. 78, 1865.

be handled without risk. By rack and pinion he was able to adjust the lens and thus the light, as required, in two directions. Cruise also differed from his predecessors in that he coated the inside of the tube with a lampblack mixture to eliminate reflections that would interfere with visualization. His light was so carefully beamed that he didn't need the bright surfaces.

Cruise's tube was introduced with a wire stylet in place. There was a fenestration near the proximal end, through which instruments might be passed. And in 1889, Cruise published the description of a means of irrigating the bladder through his scope. This was after the invention of the Nitze or Leiter-Nitze cystoscope, which Cruise thought excellent, but dangerously hot on the intravesical end.

Julius Bruck of Breslau, a dentist, conceived of lighting the object being worked on by a light source near the object to be viewed. He attempted to use a water-cooled platinum wire electrically heated to white heat. This was placed in the rectum and transilluminated the bladder. This diaphanoscopy was dangerous, and not effective, and it was dropped. In the meantime, Howard Kelly of Baltimore was using the reflected light from an otolaryngologist's head mirror to illuminate the bladder and ureteral orifices through a hollow cystoscopic speculum called the Kelly vesical speculum (Figs. 29–31). Kelly's female patients were placed in the knee-chest position. When the bladder was emptied of urine, it became filled with air and did not collapse, owing to the patient's position.

In 1847, Josef Grunfeld placed a glass window at the end of his cystoscope and passed bougies or catheters alongside the tube into the ureteral orifices under direct visual control in an aqueous or uriniferous medium. Other urologists had emptied the bladder and filled it with air in order to work inside it.

Max Nitze, an instrument maker, knew of these efforts to examine the bladder. He realized that the main problem was illumination. With an external light source the area visualized was very small, limited as it was by the internal diameter of the speculum. Dissipated by the distance from the source, the

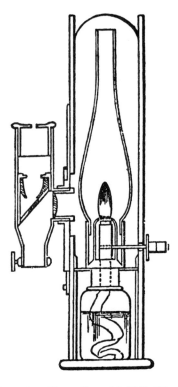

FIG. 27. *Cruise's scope. (From Fenwick EH: The Electric Illumination of the Bladder and Urethra. London, J&A Churchill, 1889.)*

light was very poor. He knew that a relatively small amount of light close to the bladder wall would be better; he sought such a source and a method of enlarging the field of vision within the bladder. According to Leo Buerger, Nitze's development of a cystoscopic lens system was a serendipitous result of checking a lens for cleanliness and seeing a clear inverted image of the church across the street.

It became clear to Nitze that by using the proper combination of lenses he could produce an enlarged field of vision, and that if the assemblage was small enough it could be moved

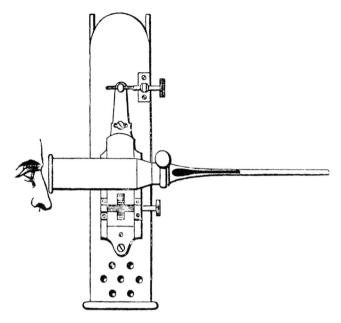

FIG. 28. *Another view of the Cruise scope. (From Fenwick EH: The Electric Illumination of the Bladder and Urethra. London, J&A Churchill, 1889.)*

throughout the bladder and used to see most of the bladder wall. Through much experimentation and many failures, he hit on using a platinum wire, heated to white heat electrically and cooled by circulating water. This was a refinement of the same method used earlier by Julius Bruck. Nitze said he wasn't aware of Bruck's work, and this may well have been so, for few at the time were aware of the attempts at diaphanoscopy and the lighting methods suggested. In an attempt to shield the bladder from the hot loop Nitze at first used a goose quill, and the loop was enclosed in glass and cooled by circulating water.

In 1877, Nitze went to Diecke, an instrument maker of Dresden who executed his ideas and fabricated the "first

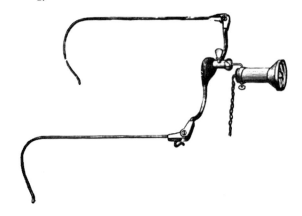

FIG. 29. *Kelly's cystoscope. The head light was used by some as a source of illumination. (From Fenwick EH: A Handbook of Clinical Cystoscopy. London, J&A Churchill, 1904.)*

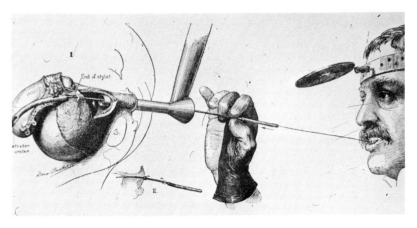

FIG. 30. *Kelly's female cystoscope in use; catheterization of a ureter under direct vision, using a head mirror and reflected light. (From Kelly HA, Burnam CF: Diseases of the Kidneys, Ureters and Bladder. Vol I, New York City, Appleton, 1914.)*

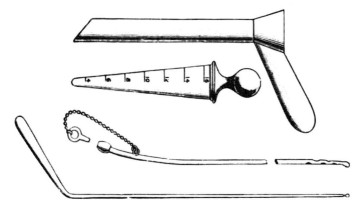

FIG. 31. *Kelly's instruments for female cystoscopy. (From Fenwick EH: A Handbook of Clinical Cystoscopy. London, J&A Churchill, 1904.)*

cystoscope." It placed the light close to the field to be examined and used lenses and an electrically heated platinum loop. This was a large bulky instrument, water-cooled, and not actually very practical because the wire loop was always dangerously close to causing terrible burns of the bladder and urethra and it burned out frequently. So Nitze and Diecke had designed and made their first direct-vision instrument, but Diecke lacked sufficient technical and mechanical experience to further perfect the instrument as Nitze wanted it. Nitze then took his idea to Leiter, an excellent and well-known instrument maker of Vienna.

In 1879, the Nitze–Leiter cystoscope was presented (Fig. 32). Leiter was a very skilled instrument maker, and the instrument was very cleverly made. It was manufactured with concave and convex sheaths. The platinum loop was still the light source, and it was now placed behind a quartz shield and water cooled. The instrument was fitted with a mandrin or occlusive obturator which, when the scope had been introduced, was removed and the urine allowed to flow from the bladder. The bladder then could be irrigated or filled with air

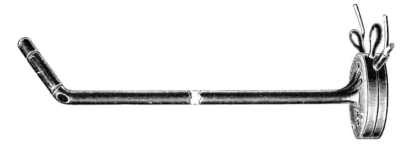

FIG. 32. *Nitze—Leiter cystoscope, the first electrically illuminated instrument. (From Fenwick, EH: A Handbook of Clinical Electric Light Cystoscopy. London, J&A Churchill, 1914.)*

or water for examination, after which the telescope was inserted into the sheath. The second instrument was a big improvement, because a prism was inserted near the fenestration and the visual field was angulated 45 degrees. In order to better illuminate this new field, the light was moved into the angulated tip and the fenestration was made on the concave surface so the examination could be much more complete. It was still bulky, unreliable, and difficult to manufacture. The electrical apparatus was poorly developed, the old batteries fumed considerably, and the rheostats were frequently unreliable.

The cystoscope was known and understood, but not widely accepted until after Thomas Edison invented the electric lamp. In 1880, Edison invented the incandescent lamp, and the inside, closed-off world of the bladder eventually opened up as a result of its use in cystoscopes.

David Newman of Glasgow was the first to use Edison's electric lamp with a cystoscope (Figs. 33–35) . His scope was of the direct-vision type with a glass on the end. The lamp was passed into the bladder separately, as were ureteral catheters or any other instruments. This instrument was large in caliber and was of no use in males.

In 1887, two men independently placed Edison's lamp at

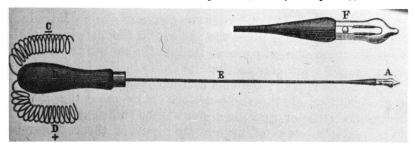

FIG. 33. *Newman's cystoscope, one of the first to use the electric lamp. (From Newman D: Lectures to Practitioners on the Diseases of the Kidney Amenable to Surgical Treatment. London, Longmans, 1888.)*

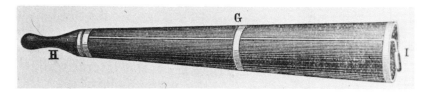

FIG. 34. *Speculum of the Newman cystoscope, with cover (to protect glass disc and facilitate introduction) in position, ready for introduction into bladder. (From Newman D: Lectures to Practitioners on the Diseases of the Kidney Amenable to Surgical Treatment. London, Longmans, 1888.)*

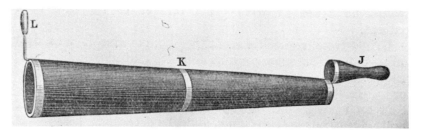

FIG. 35. *The cover (J) of Newman's cystoscope, rotated by handle (L). In position after it has been introduced into bladder. (From Newman D: Lectures to Practitioners on the Diseases of the Kidney Amenable to Surgical Treatment. London, Longmans, 1888.)*

the end of Nitze's scope. Hartwig, of Berlin, and Leiter both produced very similar instruments. The cooling system was no longer needed and the optical system could now be enlarged, giving a much larger visual field and much better visualization with the added light available. Nitze's ideas of a distal light source and an optical system for enlargement and clarification revolutionized endoscopy, let alone cystoscopy. It is of interest that Nitze's addition of the prism, which made the improved angulated vista a reality, also inverted the image seen by the urologist in these indirect instruments.

The mignon lamp, a low-amperage small bright light, was the forerunner of the next change in cystoscopes. This was invented in 1898 in Rochester, New York, by Charles Preston, and it was soon used in most endoscopic instruments. The cystoscope could now be smaller in caliber and much more readily passed.

In 1899, F. Tilden Brown attached two catheterizing channels to the lens system and showed for the first time his single-sheath system with the light in the tip of the sheath. He used two separate lens systems to see all parts of the bladder using direct and indirect methods. The same sheath was used for both lens systems, so the patient was instrumented only once. The irrigating channels were an advancement but not actually adequate for aspirations of particulate matter after litholapaxy. Therefore, Leo Buerger later modified Brown's scope further by adding several separate sheaths and telescopes, each for a specific use. This became the Brown–Buerger cystoscope, almost universally used in the United States at this time.

Leopold Dittel also placed the bulb at the end of the beak instead of within it. This made it practical to see much more of the bladder at one time with one instrument. In 1887, cystoscopy was in more general use among urologists.

In 1885, Boisseau du Rocher had presented a megaloscope, with a large field of vision. Not too different from all the earlier cystoscopes, the most important contribution of his instrument was a large sheath through which a large lens system could be inserted, still leaving room for two channels in the sheath through which the user could irrigate the bladder or even pass two ureteral catheters (Fig. 36). This was probably the greatest single contribution to the cystoscope since that of Nitze. Alexander Brenner also added a small tube to the shaft of his instrument, and he used this for irrigation or single catheterization in the male. Although Gustav Simon had passed a ureteral catheter through the urethra of a female and into the ureteral orifice on his finger and thus blindly catheterized the ureter many years before (Fig. 20), catheterization of the male ureter was actually first done by F. Tilden Brown of Baltimore.

It had been thought sufficient to see into the bladder with these instruments, without the capability of passing catheters or other instruments. Now attention and effort were given to better instrumentation and manipulation.

Because the irrigating channels were no longer needed to cool the light source, Nitze now developed an instrument with a channel that could be moved forward and backward when in the bladder, thus placing the catheter tip near the desired orifice (Fig. 37).

Leopold Casper invented a single catheterizing instrument with a removable outer wall in the catheterizing sheath (Fig. 38). After the first catheter was passed up a ureter, the wall was removed and the catheter pushed out of the sheath. When the wall was replaced, leaving one catheter outside the sheath,

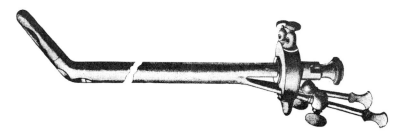

FIG. 36. *Megaloscope of Boisseau du Rocher. (From Casper Leopold: Lehrbuch der Urologie. Berlin, Urban & Schwarzenburg, 1923.)*

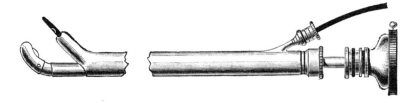

FIG. 37. *Nitze's male catheterizing cystoscope. The catheter was aimed at the ureteral orifice by moving the outer sheath. (From Fenwick EH: A Handbook of Clinical Cystoscopy. London, J&A Churchill 1904.)*

a second catheter was passed in the now empty channel. The first catheter-deflecting cystoscope was probably this one devised by Casper. In Casper's instrument, the catheter was made to lie in a groove on the ventral or concave surface and was covered by the sliding section of the sheath. This sliding segment was narrow and movable by a gentle motion at the other end of the scope. By slightly retracting this cover, the catheter could emerge over more of an angle; by advancing it, the catheter was moved in a straight-ahead direction. This indirect manipulation of the catheter was later replaced by the superior mechanism of Albarran.

Joaquin Albarran added to the Nitze cystoscope a direct method for deflecting and directing the catheter. By means of a lateral thrumbscrew, a small lid or deflector could be elevated or depressed, correspondingly elevating or depressing the catheter at its point of emergence. At first this device was separate from the scope and clamped on; later it was fused to the shaft.

About 1900, Reinhold Wappler set up a medicoelectric shop. He had arrived in America ten years before and was working with medical electric instruments for therapy, electrolysis, nerve testing, and other diagnostic procedures.

Urologists using the earliest cystoscopes and endoscopes had to obtain them from Germany, where Leiter and Wolff, among others, made these scopes. They also had to ship them

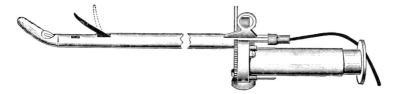

FIG. 38. *Casper's male catheterizing cystoscope. (From Fenwick HE: A Handbook of Clinical Cystoscopy. London, J&A Churchill, 1904.)*

back to Germany for repairs when needed. These instruments were far from the efficient ones we have now; they developed leaks and short circuits, and the lenses shifted. The instruments spent much of their time traveling back and forth to Germany. Repairs might well take six months to a year, from the time they were shipped out until their return through customs.

Ferdinand C. Valentine, M.D., a New York urologist, enlisted the aid of Wappler to help repair his instruments. This enabled Valentine to work without interruption. He was loud and lavish in praising Wappler's know-how and skills. Because of Valentine's praise and the obvious need for such a service, Wappler set himself up in business, forming the Wappler Electric Co., which eventually became American Cystoscope Makers, Inc. He began by copying, but he soon exceeded the originators in making cystoscopes.

William K. Otis, M.D., another urologist, stated:

Some six or seven years ago it was impossible to have disabled cystoscopes repaired in this country, and the necessity of sending them abroad for this purpose was often a decided inconvenience. About this time I was fortunate enough to make the acquaintance of Mr. Reinhold Wappler, a most skillful electrician who had already acquired an enviable reputation for the manufacture of electromedical instruments, and together we began a series of experiments in the attempt to develop the possibilities of the cystoscope.

Wappler, in an autobiographic sketch left for his family, says:

Intensely interested in catheterizing cystoscopes and for operation was Dr. F. Tilden Brown. He was untiring in his efforts to make improvements. Also Dr. Hugh H. Young of the Brady Institute in Baltimore gave specifications which tended to make the American products superior to the German make.

Brown presented what was probably the first double-catheterizing cystoscope in May of 1900. This was a modification of the Brenner single-catheterizing scope. Synchronous catheterization was now comparatively easy, and the diagnostic data became much more valuable. As Brown said then:* "In the future, any device which does not provide for such synchronous collection as a routine measure must be considered antiquated." Within a year, both Nitze and Casper had changed their cystoscopes from single- to double-catheter instruments.

Many other urologists came to Wappler, who with his brother, was now the most important producer of endoscopes of all sorts in the United States. Because Wappler was almost the only manufacturer of cystoscopes in the United States, all new inventions were of necessity funneled through the Wappler plant. Some urologists came to the Wapplers with "original ideas," only to find that others had preceded them with similar ideas. This sometimes caused bad feelings, resulting on several occasions in bitter feuds between urologists.

In 1900, Hugh Young suggested a double-prism system for a retrospective lens; in 1902 Bierhoff devised an instrument that would enable the catheterization of both ureters and then the withdrawal of the instrument, leaving the catheters in the ureters. In 1905, William K. Otis, working with Reinhold Wappler, presented a new lens system for the telescope. The prisms were replaced with hemispheric plano lenses, and the

---

* Brown FT: *Transactions of the American Association of Genitourinary Surgeons* 2:371, 1907.

wide-angle lens cystoscope was invented. A short beak and obtuse angle were used, enabling better manipulation both in men and women. This was later the basis for the Buerger instrument. It also ended inversion of the image and enabled the urologist to see the inside of the bladder in true proportion and position.

Bransford Lewis developed a number of instruments that could be manipulated through the cystocope, such as forceps, scissors, and dilators. This was the beginning of the cystoscopic attack on ureteral stones, stricture, and ureteroceles. In 1906, the Bransford Lewis Universal scope was introduced. It had a fenestration on both the convex and concave surfaces for illumination and observation on both sides. Young's retrograde lens was also used. This was, then, a complete instrument that could be used for all the purposes that the modern instrument can be used. Most modern cystoscopes, with the exception of the McCarthy panendoscope, or as it was known, the "cystourethroscope," have been built with the Universal cystoscope of Lewis as a basic model.

Leo Buerger, a fine urologist and student of cystoscopes and cystoscopy, developed his own instrument, later called the Brown–Buerger combination cystoscope. It consisted of concave and convex sheaths; observation, double-catheterizing, and operating lenses; and an obturator. The cystoscope had come of age.

Because Brown had emphasized the value of the separate-sheath principle in the United States, Buerger requested that the new instrument be named the Brown–Buerger.

Reinhold Wappler, called by Leo Buerger "the mechanical genius without whose aid the apparatus would not have attained its perfected state," described this new system in his autobiographic papers:

This instrument, devised in 1906 and introduced to the profession in 1907, is now accepted by practically all genitourinary surgeons and urologists as being the standard cystoscope for examination of the interior of the bladder and ureteral catheterization, as well as high-frequency current application. Since its introduction numerous improvements have been made in technical detail and construction of the optical system, so that we have today a catheterizing telescope which gives an upright image, a larger field, and many times more light than has been possible heretofore.

Development of X-ray Studies

In 1895, the discovery of x rays by Roentgen set off a rush by specialists of all kinds to use this new diagnostic method in their fields. However, not all the various organs were visible by means of these new rays. In order to see kidneys, ureters, and bladder, it soon became obvious that something must be put into them in order to delineate their outlines.

Urologists jumped to this effort and tried many different ways to visualize the urinary tract. Marin-Théodore Tuffier, in 1897, used a catheter up a ureter with a stylet or mandrin of metal remaining in the catheter. The metal, of course, could readily be seen by the as yet imperfected x-rays; thus, the general course of the ureter could be estimated. Radiopaque stones could be picked up if they were large enough and sufficiently dense, but urologists badly needed a more accurate way to diagnose diseases of the urinary tract. Many urologists used wires, leaded catheters, and metal-painted catheters to delineate ureters, all inadequate. To quote Edward L. Keyes:* "Painted catheters give an uncertain shadow," and

* Keyes EL: Radiographic studies in the renal pelvis and ureter. *Trans Am Urol Assoc* 3:351–357, 1909–10.

catheters with stylets have "the disadvantage of distorting the true relations of the ureter because of the stiffness of the wire."

In 1910, A. A. Uhle and G. E. Pfahler* published in the *Annals of Surgery* the suggestion that "catheters be filled with bismuth paste, metal stylets, or fluids of sufficient density to cast a shadow." B. Klose, who in 1904 had shown a case of double ureter by using two styleted catheters, suggested injecting bismuth into the pelvis and ureter through a catheter, but he didn't try it. Keller (1904) used air as an opaque medium; filling a bladder with air, he was able to demonstrate a diverticulum. Wolff went further in diagnostic methodology by injecting a suspension of 10 percent bismuth and subnitrate into the bladder.

Fritz Voelcker and Alexander von Lichtenberg used two percent collargol, a silver solution, for cystography; in 1906, they injected the same material in a retrograde manner up a catheter into the renal pelvis, thereby effecting the first pyelography. They had outlined the renal pelvis and calyces in an x ray for the first time in man. Other urologists tried other stronger silver solutions. Argyrol and five percent silver iodide emulsions were used in the kidney and ureter. These solutions were highly toxic to the urothelium and kidneys were damaged; deaths resulted from these first attempts. Animal experiments showed the damage done by these silver solutions to the kidneys. Owing to precipitation of the proteins, great damage resulted. Some, like Daniel Eisendrath, thought the severe damage was due to overinjection by volume and the introduction of silver into the circulation. Some thought it due to injection under too much pressure, and others thought the trouble due to the material injected. Actually, it was probably all these things together.

It was obvious that a liquid suitable for retrograde pyelography must first be radiopaque—it must cast a shadow in the roentgenogram. It must be nontoxic, nonirritating, and suffi-

* Uhle AA, Pfahler GE: Combined cystoscopic and roentgenographic examination of the kidneys and ureter. *Ann Surg 51*:546–551, 1910.

ciently fluid to pass out with the urine, leaving no residue. Bismuth preparations were mostly insoluble and precipitated too rapidly. Bismuth salts were toxic, and limewater was not radiopaque. Silver salts irritated the mucosa and were very messy to work with, staining everything with which they came in contact. Five percent silver iodide was found to be antiseptic, bland, and gave a good x-ray shadow. Thorium nitrate-citrate also worked well, but it gave off gamma radiation and irritative phenomena were noted. It also was a good culture medium for molds and became toxic after standing for a time. With all its drawbacks, thorium nitrate-citrate was used for years until 1918, when D. F. Cameron brought out a mixture of sodium and potassium iodide. The potassium was soon taken out of this mixture because of its toxicity. Sodium iodide (13.5 percent) was found to be excellent and to have low toxicity; it was isotonic with urine and gave good x-ray films.

Many media and methods were given up for good and sufficient reasons. Among these were use of air and carbon dioxide because they were hard to differentiate from bowel gases; additionally, the danger of air emboli could not be dismissed. Umkrenal and lithium iodide were too expensive and irritating; lipiodol was oily and failed to mix with urine. Umbrathor and colloidal thorium dioxide were too viscid, causing irritation and obstruction. Umbrathor was fine in the bladder and was freely used for cystograms; unfortunately it was absorbed by the reticuloendothelial system, causing cellular damage. Another little known method for studying kidney morphology was injection of material into the peritoneum. Air, oxygen, and carbon dioxide were all used and information with regard to size, shape, and location of the kidneys sometimes resulted.

But x-rays were still not sharply delineated until the introduction of the Bucky moving grid. This great advance increased the sharpness of the film, and it also increased the field of useful shadows. The x-ray film thus could be used to visualize the entire genitourinary tract. Films were again improved when double coating and double intensification were added. In addition, the tables used for genitourinary roentgenography were improved to enable positional changes. The time was right for further efforts to delineate the kidneys and ureters roentgenographically.

Many different means of attack were outlined, many attempted, and some used for more than just experimentation. Pericystic and perirenal pneumoradiography consisted of injecting oxygen, carbon dioxide, or air into the spaces around the kidney and bladder. The dangers of infection and of embolization were always present, and the x-ray techniques used at that time did not result in much helpful diagnostic information. Pneumoradiography was thus abandoned until fairly recently.

Pneumoperitoneum was supposed to be helpful in differentiating intra- and extraperitoneal masses; the dangers attached to that procedure are obvious. Its use did not last long. Attempts were also made to coat nonopaque calculi with collargol or lipiodol and then x-ray them. This, too, proved less than satisfactory.

Arteriography (actually aortography) was introduced early in the development of these tests by Santos. He suggested injecting iodide solution into the aorta. This was done by direct percutaneous injection with the patient under anesthesia. The material used was an iodide solution and was used to outline the abdominal vessels, such as the renal arteries. But this was considered too dangerous and also superfluous because it could not help in diagnosis. Our modern angiograms are derivatives of this first daring maneuver. Seminal vesiculography also was first tried in those early days, but it was not found very helpful. We still use it too sparingly.

Two well-known tests have been handed down practically unchanged as valuable additions to our diagnostic armamentarium. Cystourethrography is the use of a contrast material to fill and outline the bladder, sometimes also outlining contents such as stones or tumors, resulting in easily seen filling defects. Reflux may also become obvious. Films are taken during voiding, and this sometimes identifies urethral lesions and high-pressure reflux.

The second method is retrograde ureteropyelography—the injection into the kidneys and the ureters of radiopaque material through a ureteral catheter. For both tests sodium iodides, potassium iodides, or iodized oils were usually the materials of choice until a short time later when the organic iodides were introduced.

The introduction and use of organic iodides led to perhaps the single greatest invention in urologic diagnosis—the intravenous urogram. Although ureteral catheterization was useful and retrograde pyelography proved greatly enlightening, many difficulties and dangers were still associated with this technique. Thus, the search continued for a material that could be injected intravenously, concentrated in, and excreted by the kidneys, yet was still radiopaque and harmless to the tissues.

Leonard G. Rowntree, in 1923, used 10 percent solution of sodium iodide intravenously and by mouth. With this, he and his co-workers were usually able to visualize the bladder and, in some cases, the renal pelvis and ureter. In the following year, Paul Rosenstein and von Lichtenberg repeated this work in conjunction with perirenal pneumoradiography. Volkmann used various halogen compounds and settled on 10 percent sodium iodide. Theodor Hrynstschak and others all used some of these materials, but found that quantities sufficiently large to give good visualization of the kidneys were too dangerous to the patient.

In 1928, Professor A. Roseno was trying iodides and urea, a mixture later called pyelognost. Visualization of the kidney was recognized by Roseno as a new diagnostic aid and many patients were injected with this material for urologic diagnosis. Severe reactions, large dosage, and only fair visualization of the urinary collecting systems made this material unsatisfactory.

In 1929, an organically bound iodide known as uroselectan or iopax was introduced by Moses Swick, M.D., of New York

City. Because the facts of the introduction of this important drug have sometimes been confused by historians, the following outline was obtained directly from Dr. Swick.

As a young man, Swick studied and performed research in Germany. He started in the Hamburg laboratory of Professor Lichtwitz, where experimentation with a drug used to combat animal infections was going on. This drug—selectan neutral—was originated by Karl Binz, a chemist working at a veterinary college laboratory in Berlin. It was an iodide compound, and the halogens in various compounds were known to be radiopaque. When they began using the drug on man as an agent to combat infections, Swick tried it for urography as well. When 7.5 gm of selectan neutral was injected intravenously, it caused headache, nausea, and double vision, but it did produce faint, vague pyelograms.

Swick went back to Binz and requested a similar but less toxic compound. Binz produced another double iodo compound, but it was insoluble and of course was not helpful in intravenous urography. Another was only eight percent soluble—still insufficient. By this time, it became obvious to Swick that he should make himself more readily available to Binz, so he moved his work to the laboratories of Professor von Lichtenberg in Berlin, where Binz was working.

Swick and Binz then reduced the drug to a monoiodo form by eliminating one of the iodine atoms. This material was 42 percent soluble and proved to be nontoxic in dogs, rabbits, and finally humans. In June of 1929, von Lichtenberg was in the United States at a meeting of the A.U.A. when Swick, though a third party, informed von Lichtenberg of his success. Von Lichtenberg spoke of this upcoming breakthrough as if it were his own, and so was acclaimed by many in the United States as its originator. In fact, von Lichtenberg scheduled a paper to be presented that fall discussing the origins and use of uroselectan; the authors were given as von Lichtenberg and Swick. Swick protested and at a meeting with all the participants it was decided that Swick would speak first on the medical breakthrough, its origins, background, and chemistry, to be followed by von Lichtenberg discussing the clinical use.

At the next annual A.U.A. meeting Swick was barred from presenting his most important paper, whereas von Lichtenberg was an invited speaker. To this date, many urologists do not know that Moses Swick was the sole originator and developer of our most important radiologic diagnostic tool—the intravenous urogram.

From this discovery grew modern urologic diagnosis. Intravenous urography first, then tomography, aortography, and angiography all resulted from the findings of a material intravenously injected and concentrated and excreted by the kidneys, and casting a dense x-ray shadow.

Gonorrhea and Syphilis

The term *gonorrhea* in Greek means "a flow of offspring—a flow of semen." Galen may have been the first to so name it, thinking that the purulent discharge was a leakage of semen. Many have made attempts to change the name, as it obviously does not correctly identify the discharge or point in any way to the origin of the disease. *Blennorrhea* was one term suggested for its name; this also was inept, meaning "mucus flow." Other terms have been mentioned but *gonorrhea* has stuck. Such slang terms as *clap, woman's disease,* and *chaude–pisse* (hot urine) have been used for years and are readily understood by all affected. *Clap* was a name probably derived from the red-light district in Paris, known as "Le Clapier," and the houses known as "clapise."

Urethritis was mentioned in the Bible, in the Egyptian papyruses, and in all the early Hindu literature. Hippocrates knew of it and mentioned the suppuration and flow of pus seen in the disease. Aristotle and Plato described what undoubtedly must have been gonorrhea. Epicurus developed a postgonorrheal stricture and committed suicide while in urinary retention.

Galen called this purulent urethritis by its now commonly

accepted misnomer, *gonorrhea*. His therapy consisted of anti-phlogistines—literally, "against inflammation."

The Mesopotamian tablets and also some of the Samhitas and other early sources discuss what we must presume to have been gonorrhea: "If a man's penis on occasions of his pleasure hurts him, boil beer and milk and anoint him from his pubis." Another therapeutic measure described:

> If a man's urine is like the urine of an ass, like beer yeast, like wine yeast or varnish, that man is sick of gonorrhea and through a bronze tube in the penis pour oil and beer and licorice. . . . If a man in his sleep or in his walking has seminal discharge and his penis and his clothes are full of seminal fluid, thou shalt mix in oil, clay of the dust of the mountain stone and horned alkali. Thou shalt smear a plaster on the point of the man's tongue and in oil and wine thou shalt mix it. He shall drink it and he will recover.

Also passages are found such as: "If a man's urine is like the urine of an ass, that man is sick of gonorrhea; if a man's urine is like varnish, that man is sick of gonorrhea." "If a man discharges blood from his penis like a woman," and other similar passages describe what was undoubtedly gonorrhea.

Many means of treatment have been advised over the intervening years. Galen used antiphlogistines; Avicenna suggested placing a louse in the urethra as a sort of counterirritant maneuver; Constantinus was said to have suggested a soothing injection of milk. More soothing were the balms later advised. Incidentally, the Bible suggests that a man remain away from woman for 14 days after his discharge has dried up.

Before the sixteenth century, gonorrhea and syphilis were known as separate diseases, until a group called the Identists claimed they were one and the same and interchangeable. John Hunter, a man held in very high esteem, inoculated himself with matter from a disease he thought was only gonorrhea and found he had both syphilis and gonorrhea. This proved to him that they were one and the same, with different symptoms. His dictum about this remained the rule for 100 years.

Benjamin Bell, with the assistance of some volunteers and medical students—obviously unafraid of lues or gonorrhea in those heroic days before antibiotics—made efforts to disprove the Hunterian pronouncements. Bell quotes from his students' reports:*

Matter was taken upon the point of a probe from a chancre on the glans penis, before any application was made to it, and completely introduced into the urethra, expecting thereby to produce gonorrhea. For the first eight days, I felt no kind of uneasiness, but about this period I was attacked with pain in passing water. On dilating the urethra as much as possible, nearly the whole of a large chancre was discovered, and in a few days thereafter, a bubo was formed in each groin. No discharge took place from the urethra during the whole course of the disease. Mercury, in the form of mercurial ointment was rubbed in the outside of each thigh and the buboes and chancres finally healed.

Venereal infection, that bitter scourge of unlawful embraces, would have proved the reproach of physicians had not 'quick-silver' happily been found to be its antidote.

Lastly, it may not be amiss to admonish that the most proper time for ordering a salivation is either when pocky eruptions have for some time appeared on the body, or when ulcers appear, especially in the mouth and throat.†

Mercury was, of course, the cure for syphilis.

Bell continues: "The next experiment was made with the matter of gonorrhea, a portion of which was introduced between the prepuce and glans and allowed to remain there without being disturbed. In the course of the second day, a slight degree of inflammation was produced, succeeded by a discharge of matter, which, in the course of two or three days, disappeared." Imagine the presumption! "The same experiment was, by the same gentleman, repeated once again, after

* Bell Benjamin: *A Treatise on Gonorrhea Virulenta and Lues Venerea.* Vol I, Philadelphia. Printed for Robert Campbell, bookseller, 1795.

† Mead Richard: *Medical Precepts and Cautions.* Translated by Thomas Stack Dublin, Printed for W Smith at Hercules in Dame Street, 1751.

rendering the parts tender to which the matter of gonorrhea was applied; but no chancre ever ensued from it."

Bell then goes on to say that "two young gentlemen, while prosecuting the study of medicine became anxious to ascertain the point in question . . ." The two young men inoculated themselves with "matter from gonorrhea." They expected chancres, but both developed severe gonorrhea, and no chancres ensued. One developed such a severe case that

. . . nor did he for upwards of a year get entirely free from it. By this he was convinced of the imprudence and hazard of all such experiments, nor could he be prevailed on to carry them farther, although they were keenly prosecuted by his friend, who, soon after the inflammation arising from his first experiment was removed, inserted the matter of gonorrhea on the point of a lancet beneath the skin of the preputium, and likewise into the substance of the glans, but *although this was repeated three different times,* no chancres ensued. . . . His last experiment was attended with more serious consequences. The matter of a chancre was inserted on the point of a probe to the depth of a quarter of an inch, or more, in the urethra. No symptoms of gonorrhea ensued, but . . . chancre was perceived and bubos and ulcers of the throat . . . nore was a cure obtained till a very large quantity of mercury was given under a state of close confinement for a period of thirteen weeks.

These unnamed, unafraid gentlemen—medical students and scientists—did much to disprove the theory of the Identists and showed "that there is a very strong presumption that, at least in the great majority of cases, the poison of gonorrhea is not identical with that of chancre." The good Doctor Bell was not one to go out on a limb.

In 1859, F.J. Bumstead summarized in his *A Treatise on the Veneral Disease* as follows:*

Hunter inoculated gonorrheal pus and produced a chancre, followed by its characteristic constitutional symptoms. Harrison conveyed pus

* *A Treatise on the Veneral Disease* by John Hunter, FRS, with copious additions by Dr. Philip Ricord, Ed 2, Translated and edited by Freeman J Bumstead. Philadelphia, Blanchard and Lea, 1859.

from a chancre, by means of a sound, into the urethra, and produced a gonorrhea; when it has been concluded that the cause of these two is identical . . . Tode, Duncan, as well as Bell in his experiments, have never succeeded in producing a chancre with gonorrheal matter, while pus from a chancre introduced into the urethra was followed by a chancre in that canal; which facts have of necessity, led them to admit a difference in the intimate nature of the two diseases. And yet, all these experiments are true, although contradictory, for their difference is only apparent and dependent upon an erroneous interpretation.

Bumstead's book goes on to draw some correct interpretations about chancres. Whenever matter produced chancres unsuspectedly, chancres must have at one time been present, although unsuspected or undiagnosed at that time. Philippe Ricord was probably the most famous proponent of the different origins and different identities of the two diseases. He was also quite a humorist, as evidenced by an anecdote in a personal communication from Dr. Adrian Zorgniotti. On one occasion, while tending wounded soldiers under fire in France, a passing officer sent a messenger to tell him "to withdraw before he received a bullet." The doctor is said to have replied: "I am not receiving today, as I am not in my office."

M. Vidal was a proponent of the single-identity theory of venereal disease. He stated that gonorrhea and syphilis are due to a specific virus, and nonvirulent gonorrhea differs. Vidal's arguments fell flat when he attempted to differentiate specific gonorrhea from other types: "It is difficult to distinguish the two, but if you can satisfy yourself that there was a true incubation in the case, and if the discharge tends to a chronic state, you will incline to believe it specific, and vice versa, and if syphilitic symptoms afterwards appear, the diagnosis will be plain." I have recently heard similar obfuscated statements from politicians seeking office.

In 1838, Philippe Ricord inoculated 667 persons with gonorrhea and failed completely to produce syphilis. This was an autoinoculation program in which matter from discharge was inoculated into another skin location. He differentiated between a veneral ulceration and gonorrhea, but not between chancre and syphilis. Ricord held that gonorrhea was a simple inflammation brought on by various viruses, and syphilis was caused by another specific virus. Ricord is also credited with the oft-quoted statement that "Paris is the capital of the syphilized world." Not until 1872 did Haller discover microorganisms in the pus of gonorrhea; in 1879, Albert Neisser discovered and described the gonococcus and proved this to be the causative organism of the urethral and ocular gonorrhea. Somewhat later, Ernst Finger studied the pathophysiology of gonorrhea and proved the organisms were penetrating far below the mucosa and around the glands of Littre and of Morgagni. P. S. Pelouze's study and awareness of this pathology led to his new dictum of "gentle care."

The care or therapy of gonorrhea took many steps in the early 1900s: vaccines, digested gonococcus solutions, nonspecific proteins for a febrile reaction to cure, and then specific drugs. Acriflavine was suggested in 1917, and Hugh Young proposed Mercurochrome in 1918. Postassium permanganate —"the purple passion plunge"—was another solution used. These were usually injected directly into the urethra, and if handling was not gentle, posterior urethritis, prostatitis, and other spread of the infection resulted. Pelouze suggested gonophage—a parallel to bacteriophage—in 1927. The next great step forward—the one that emptied the heretofore heavily occupied hospital wards given over to pelvic inflammatory disease (usually gonorrhea), and did the most to prevent gonorrheal strictures—was the discovery and widespread use of the sulfa drugs in the late 1930s and early 1940s. Soon the statement "gonorrhea is no worse than a bad cold" became popular, although still most untrue. The gleet remained as a sad reminder to many too many. As Mead noted in 1751:*

* Mead Richard: *Medical Precepts and Cautions.* Translated by Thomas Stack Dublin, Printed for W Smith, at the Hercules in Dame Street, and J Exshaw at the Bible on Cork-Hill, 1751.

At first that discharge of mucous humor commonly called a gleet, which sometimes succeeds a virulent gonorrhea, is very troublesome and obstinate. It proceeds both from the vesiculae seminales and the prostate gland, by the erosion of the orifices of their ducts from the acrimony of the morbid humor; and is most commonly the result of an ill judged method of curing the gonorrhea with violent cathartics which destroy the natural tone of the fibres.

Stricture is, of course, the most serious chronic resultant of gonorrhea. Stricture must be a subject of its own and is discussed in the next chapter.

Urethral Strictures

Stricture of the urethra was explored in dissection by Hunter. He determined that the urethra was a muscular organ and that the stricture resulted from a fiber or fibers becoming inordinately or permanently contracted. He described a stricture as resembling in effect a thread tied round the membrane of the canal. Charles Bell, in 1811, disproved this to his own satisfaction and found inflammation to be the cause of stricture. He found the urethra to not be a muscular organ, and so incapable of contractile movements. Yet strictures existed.

Strictures in the urethra are always the product of inflammation, and as gonorrhea is the most frequent as well as the most intense kind of inflammation to which the urethra is subject, so is it the principal cause of strictures in this canal. In fact if we should carefully interrogate those afflicted with the latter disease, we would find that they had all experienced one or more attacks of gonorrhea—that the attack preceding the stricture had lasted a long time . . .

So said Ducamp in 1827.* He believed stricture to be a result of chronic deep-seated inflammation, usually gonorrhea.

* Ducamp Théodore: *A Treatise on Retention of Urine caused by Strictures in the Urethra.* Translated by William M Herbert. New York, Samuel Wood & Sons, 1827.

Ambroise Paré thought caruncles and carnosities resulted from superfluous flesh generated at external ulcers. Others believed these lesions to be the obstructing ones in the gonorrheal urethra. However, later research proved that the carnosities and caruncles are not the cause of stricture or caused by gonorrhea directly, but they may result from the consequences of the stricture following gonorrhea.

Whatever may be the seat or nature of the stricture, the symptoms which attend it are nearly the same, or vary only in proportion to the narrowness of the passage that is left for the urine, and the duration of the disease. If the stricture be inconsiderable, the urine flows in a small twisted or bifurcated stream: the patient passes his water slowly, and suffers no other inconvenience than a slight scalding during its evacuation, with a sense of weight at the perineum, and itching along the course of the canal. The stream gradually becomes more slender and weak, the patient takes a longer time to make water, although he passes less at once; he also experiences a greater degree of micturition, so frequent and so urgent as to oblige him to rise several times in the night. The discharge of the urine can be now accomplished only by continued efforts, and is attended with acute pain, and tumefaction of the penis . . . But the difficulty of making water may arrive at a still greater height. Indeed, we sometimes meet with persons in whom the stream is so feeble that instead of being projected to a distance from the penis, it falls vertically between the legs, like the jet of a glass cutter's wheel.

This was Ducamp's description of the symptoms. He goes even further and describes overflow incontinence and retention due to stricture. His method of diagnosis is equally simple: "We may ascertain the truth by introducing a bougie into the canal: if the instrument be stopped in its progress, or tightly wedged in a particular part of the route through which it has to pass, the existence of a stricture ceases to be doubtful."

Treatment of stricture was described in the earliest papyruses and clay tablets as dilatation. Bougies, sounds, and other similar instruments have been known and used since the earliest doctors were presented with a case of stricture, and indeed the earliest doctors probably did have patients with stricture.

Bougies, the most popular of the instruments for dilatation, are still available in much the same form now as originally used. They are flexible instruments, usually solid, cylindric, and sufficiently long to pass the length of the urethra and still be manipulated. Their sizes depend on the urethra they are to distend, and their distal ends are usually rounded.

Jean Zuléma Amussat, the great French urologist of the early 1800s, recognized strictures of three types:*

1. Organic strictures—resultant from chronic inflammation of the mucous membrane of the urethra following blenorrhagia, use of astringents, contusions, masturbation, or excessive exercise on horseback.

2. Spasmodic strictures—quite rare, a spasmodic contraction of the muscular fibres which surround the portion of the urethra situated between the bulb and the prostate gland. Seen during an acute blenorrhagia or after venereal excesses.

3. Inflammatory strictures—the result of a very great afflux of blood into the spongy tissue. This state of turgescence, which is only temporary, no more constitutes, rigorously speaking, a true stricture of the canal.

The organic strictures are the important ones therapeutically, and they may be divided into four separate types:

1. Fraeni—these are slight elevations of the mucous membranes—almost always transverse and projecting but little into the stream—actually incipient strictures.

2. Valvular strictures—fraeni occupying the entire circumference of the urethra.

3. Strictures produced by the chronic swelling of the urethral mucous membrance—more frequent in old persons rather than the

---

* Amussat JZ: *Amussat's Lectures on Retention of Urine, caused by Strictures of the Urethra and on the Diseases of the Prostate.* Translated by James P Jervey, MD, edited by A Petit, MD, Philadelphia, Haswell Barrington & Haswell, 1840.

younger. Seen in those who have had several attacks of blenorrhagia and have used bougies habitually to relieve themselves of an oozing.

4. The fourth is callous stricture when acute inflammations have extended to the subadjacent tissues and pass into the chronic state. These strictures, which rarely occur in persons who have never been subjected to cauterization, are much more frequent in those upon whom the caustic has been often and too deeply applied.

"As for vegetations and fleshy excrescences, the existence of which has perhaps been denied in too absolute a manner by some authors," Amussat had never seen them "but once." He also stated that these strictures were always distal to the bulbous portion and were very frequent at the commencement of the fossa navicularis near the meatus urinarius.

"If there be diseases the remembrance of which is soon forgotten, there is no man affected by stricture who does not throughout the whole of his life recollect a complete retention of urine, and who does not preserve for him who has relieved him, some sentiment of gratitude." So said Dr. A. Petit quoting Amussat in 1840.

Urinary retention resulting from stricture was a frequent complication, much feared and revered.

The practitioner with facility in catheterization, or of inducing urination by one means or another, was always busy. Other than catheterization and prior to more forceful and more dangerous manipulations, opium given both locally and systemically, was the greatest help. The first effect of the opium was to diminish the distress the patient experiences from the bladder distension. When the desire to urinate became less overwhelming and exertions to accomplish it less severe, then perhaps relaxation permitted urination.

Amussat also used "forced injections" of tepid water up the urethra, believing that the liquid under pressure would penetrate the stricture, dislodge any obstructing mucus and permit an efflux of urine. If the injection didn't relieve retention, it at least facilitated later instrumentation.

The conical or forcing sound (a metal catheter, thick-walled, with a rather sharply pointed conical tip) was sometimes used to force an artificial passage into the bladder. It was a true puncture of the bladder through the urethra, and it was more dangerous than direct trochar puncture, as the course of the conical tip was only poorly controlled and often caused severe trauma. Use of a suprapubic and perineal punch with a trochar was much safer because it was more readily controlled. The first perineal punches were done with a bistoury (small knife), which was thrust into the perineum at the same location that Frère Jacques used for lithotomy. When urine was seen to flow, a metallic cannula was passed alongside the bistoury and bandaged into place. In 1721, Junkers may have been the first to try the trochar for this purpose, and it remained the instrument of choice for years.

To perform the perineal puncture, the patient was placed in the lithotomy position. The trochar was plunged into the perineum on the left side of the raphe, between the urethra and the tuberosity of the ischium at about an inch from the anus.

The point of the trochar should be directed at first parallel to the axis of the body, and afterwards a little within, in order to reach the inferior part of the wall of the bladder near the neck. So soon as the absence of resistance and the passage of the urine show that the instrument has penetrated into the cavity of the viscus, the trochar is withdrawn and the cannula, which must be properly fixed, is left.

These perineal approaches were also supplemented by the suprapubic methods. Aware that the distended bladder carries the peritoneum upward with it, surgeons were able to safely pass a trochar from the suprapubic approach. This became the pathway of choice for many urologists to empty the bladder in patients with urinary retention in whom catheters could not be passed. To quote Bell:*

The bladder maybe punctured above the pubis because when it is greatly distended and has risen into the abdomen, it carries the

* Bell Charles: *A System of Operative Surgery founded on the Basis of Anatomy.* Two vols, Hartford, 1816.

peritoneum with it, so that the reflection of that membrane from the pubis to the fore part of the bladder is shifted upwards, and a space is left betwixt the bone and the reflected membrane, where the trochar may pierce into the bladder without entering the sac of the peritoneum. Unless where the bladder is distended very much, it would be improper to perform the operation here.

There were many patients who were in such distress and severity of retention that their bladders ruptured into either the peritoneum—this was tantamount to death—or extraperitoneally with resultant extravasation, gangrene, and usually death.

If the bladder did not rupture, the urethra often did, and if a fistula did not result, then extravasation, gangrene, and death often did. Surgeons were aware of these sequelae from the timid treatment of strictures; they looked for them and attempted to prevent them. If a strictured urethra could not be instrumented, the surgeon passed a sound to the stricture and cut down on it; then following the urethra proximally, he would open it widely with the knife blade, thus releasing the stricture. A silver catheter could then be passed from the meatus to the bladder, and made indwelling by being "fixed in place" (Fig. 39). "In several days when the granulations shall have covered the catheter, the tract in which it lays is consolidated, the catheter may be withdrawn, and a common bougie introduced. The urine will not make its way into the perineum again, as long as the urethra is free."

Charles Bell also described removal of a segment of diseased urethra. This was treated in almost the same way, with an indwelling catheter, for about three weeks.

Caustics were widely used to treat strictures in the 1700s and early 1800s. Kali purum and argentum nitratum were the two most common caustics. Kali purum is pure potassium and argentum nitratum is silver nitrate. Both are excellent caustics, and they were handled carefully so as to "burn" only the strictured areas. "Porte caustiques" were invented to apply the agent only where desired, and the timing of the application

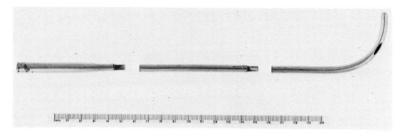

FIG. 39. *Three piece silver catheter. It could easily be carried in the pocket. (Courtesy of the Urology Museum, The Albert Einstein College of Medicine, New York City.)*

was very important. When the pain was not relieved by the application of caustic—and in those cases where the Lumen was not more distensible—sufficient cauterization either in time or in the area involved had not been effected.*

To understand the effect of caustic in subduing irritation in the urethra in cases of stricture, we may take the following conclusive example. If a man has an ulcer in the pellucid cornea of the eye, the ulcer keeps up a great deal of inflammation and irritation in the whole eye, but if we apply caustic to the bottom and tender part of this ulcer, the irritation and inflammation of the eye quickly subsides. When we examine the circumstances of this case, we find that the ulcer is highly irritable, and that the acrid tears flowing into it are a principal cause of the continance of the disorder. The touch of the caustic deadens the surface, then the tears are no longer a cause of irritation, and the general inflammation and pain therefore subside. The effect of the caustic applied to the eye in this manner is, however, only temporary; the surface touched by the caustic is thrown off and exposes a sensible granulating surface. The tears now have access to this new surface, the pain and irritation return and, to a certain degree: a second touch of the caustic again destroys the sensible surface, before it be again exposed; the hollow of the ulcer is nearly filled up, and a healthy or a more natural state of the part is substituted for the eating sore. Several such gentle applications of

* Bell Charles, *A System of Operative Surgery, founded on the Basis of Anatomy.* Two vols, Hartford, 1816.

the caustic do not prevent the ulcer from filling and a cicatrix at length forming.

The application of the caustic to the urethra has an effect very similar to this. . . . The first effect of the caustic is to destroy the sensibility, and then the urine passes without exciting spasm.

Bell actually tried the effects of these caustics on his own arm. First he removed ". . . a piece of the cuticle from my arm with the surface bled" and then he tried the caustics. He concluded, "In the way in which it is applied, it becomes a weak caustic, flowing out as it is dissolved, deadening the surface of the urethra, and subduing the inflammation, but not sufficiently powerful to bring a deep slough from the firm stricture."

Many were the injections and the remedies attempted for curing urethral discharges. Many were the discharges perpetuated by these remedies.*

Much more tolerable, and in my experience of much greater efficacy in such conditions, is the oleum santalum citrinum (oil of yellow sandalwood) . . . I have seen recovery from its use in from three to six days after the long and faithful use of injections and other internal medicines had proved unavailing. . . . A patient would now and then complain that the subject of sandalwood fans was too often introduced in his presence to be quite agreeable; beyond the odor, however, and an occasional slight dyspeptic trouble, this remedy appeared unexceptionable.

F. N. Otis thought that such discharges were not only perpetuated by stricture, but also could be caused by strictures. He used an instrument similar to the Desormeaux and Fisher endoscopes to visualize the strictures, but made specially for him out of black hard rubber. With this instrument, reflections no longer bothered him, and he was able to inspect and treat urethral lesions.

Bell sometimes found he was unable to divulse strictures

---

* Otis FN: On Chronic Urethral Discharges. (Reprinted from the *NY Med J*, June, 1870.) New York, Appleton & Co., 1870.

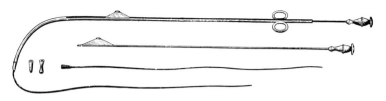

FIG. 40. *Maisonneuve's urethrotome. (From Chetwood CH: Practice of Urology, 2nd Ed, New York City, William Wood, 1916.)*

with the available instruments. All available instruments were of small caliber—Jules Maisonneuve's cutting instrument reached only 21 French (Fig. 40). Otis designed and had made his own dilating urethrotome (Fig. 41). This instrument he described as follows:

. . . a pair of straight steel bars arranged on the principle of parallel ruler, capable of expanding by means of a screw to 40 French. The upper bar is traversed by a cannula with a bulb on its end to detect strictures, as would a bougie à boule. A blade could also be inserted at a detected strictured point and utilized to incise it directly. Sufficient depth and length was obtained to divide completely strictures made tense and thin by the expansion of the dilating apparatus.

Thus the internal cutting of stricture was off to a good start.

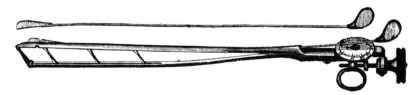

FIG. 41. *The Otis dilating urethrotome. Similar instruments are now being used by some urologists for internal urethrotomy. (From Chetwood CH: Practice of Urology. 2nd Ed, New York City, William Wood, 1916.)*

Before internal urethrotomy was done, external urethrotomy had been accomplished by many. "La boutonnière" or the button hole was a small incision in the perineum, parallel to the raphe and opening widely the urethra proximal to the structures. Indeed, it was often the best way to feel the stricture in the urethra and cut down directly upon it, opening it widely and by exposing it, hoping to permit the destruction of the stricture and opening the urethra to permit the urine to flow again. This incision may result in a fistula, but certainly this is not as bad as many of the sequelae of puncture or forced catheterization.

The Prostate: Surgical Approaches

As soon as man conquered his environment sufficiently to live long enough, his prostate became an important fact of life. Prostatism must have been the cause of many deaths in the early days. We know the Egyptians used reeds, copper and silver tubes, and rolled palm leaves to withdraw retained urine from the bladder. This may have been due to stones, prostatic obstruction, or probably both. The persons who used these instruments most, and hopefully best, became known as lithologists: the first specialists in medicine. The Hindu Vedas described cannulas of wood and metal, but they referred to stone obstructions only. The old writers described these obstructions and subsequent urinary retentions as due to excrescences and carnosities at the bladder neck. Herophilus of Chalcedon about 300 BC gave us what is probably the earliest gross description of the prostate in his anatomic texts, and Rufus of Ephesus described the parastatus glandulus. From this term, meaning "standing before" or "standing beside," prostate probably evolved.

Aristotle used the term *varicose parastatae* for what may

well have been seminal vesicles. What Rufus mentioned as *glandulosae parastatae,* may well have been the epididymis. The prostate's importance and relation to urination and procreation were not well understood then, or now.

At about the beginning of the Christian era, Aulus Cornelius Celsus (25 BC to 50 AD) described catheterization and urethrotomy in the following passage translated by G. F. Collier, M.D.:*

Circumstances sometimes render it necessary to draw off the urine by an operation; as in retention, or when the urethra has become collapsed from old age, or when a calculus or grumous blood has produced internal obstruction; so, also, even a moderate degree of inflammation often prevents natural micturition. Now this operation is necessary not only in males, but sometimes in females, also. Hence copper catheters are made for this purpose; and that they may serve for all sorts of cases, the practitioner should keep by him three for men, and two for females; the largest of the male catheters being fifteen digits, those of middle size, twelve, and the smallest nine; while of the female, the larger should be nine, and the smaller six. They ought to be somewhat curved, but the male more especially, very smooth, and of a moderate diameter. The patient is to be placed on his back, as described for operation at the anus, upon a stool or a couch. The physician standing at his right side should, in the male subjects, lay hold of the penis with his left hand, while with his right he passes the catheter into the urethra; when he has reached the neck of the bladder, he is to give the instrument, together with the penis, a slight inclination downwards, and to push it on into the bladder itself, and to withdraw it after the urine has been evacuated. In females, the urethra is shorter and straighter than the male, its nipple-like orifice being situated between the labia and above the vagina; and they also, as frequently require this kind of aid, although with them it is attended with less difficulty.

The carnosities or caruncles of the bladder neck which caused urinary obstruction and retention were treated as strictures by some early lithologists. Caustic solutions were used to

* Collier GF: *A Translation of the Eight Books of Aulus Cornelius Celsus on Medicine.* Ed 2, London, 1831.

attempt to destroy them. Unfortunately these often caused more problems than they cured, since their use was uncontrolled. Solid caustics were used in specially protected "porte caustiques," so that hopefully they would burn only the area of the stricture. These were hollow rods with caustic-soaked lint applicators to be pushed forward at the stricture or hollow rods with applicators with cups for solid caustic materials that could be used for one side or another directionally at the will of the operator (Fig. 42). Other metallic rods with windows were used in attempts to curette the obstructing tissues (Fig. 43).

Other surgeons filed ridges in sounds about an inch behind the tip. These would be passed through the obstructed area, pulled back and forth, and also twisted, probably removing some of the excrescences and carnosities. All methods used undoubtably gave some relief. Ambroise Paré invented an instrument to destroy carnosities by cutting (Fig. 44). This was actually a forerunner of the modern resectroscope.

Tunneling through the prostate was also an accepted therapy; this was usually done transurethrally and consisted of the "forced catheterization" method. A metal catheter with a rather sharp conical point was passed easily to the obstruction, and then forced upward into the bladder, usually through the midportion of the prostate. A catheter was then left indwelling for a short time (several days). After its removal, the patient voided through the newly made tunnel, with or without control.

Cystotomy, generally perineal, was in widespread use for the removal of stones. It was obvious that this would also receive obstruction due to the prostate. Sometimes it was necessary to remove portions of the prostate to obtain access to the stone. Thus, the first prostatic surgery was probably unintentional and through a perineal approach. Suprapubic cystotomy was tried in the 1550s, but it did not become popular until after anatomist John Hunter had shown that the distended bladder carried the peritoneum upward out of the pelvis, making it possible to open the bladder without entering the peritoneum.

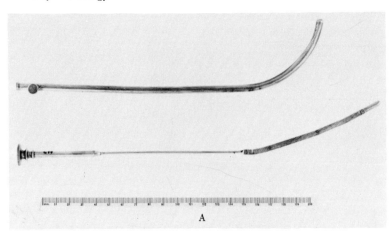

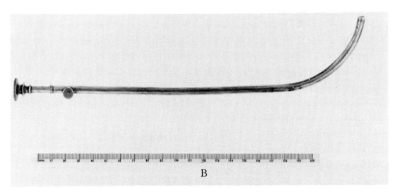

FIG. 42. *Instrument used to carry cauterization materials such as silver nitrate to ulcers or strictures. A, Disassembled. B, Assembled, ready for use. (Courtesy of the Urology Museum, Albert Einstein College of Medicine, New York City.)*

Perineal prostatic resection done with the bistoury blade was accomplished in 1639 unknowingly by Joseph Covillard, and others carried out similar procedures in the following years. This was merely the surgical excision of a wedge or nubbin of tissue to enable urine to pass. Total prostatectomy

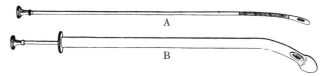

FIG. 43. *Leroy d'Étiolles' instrument for lateral retrograde cauterization. A, The cannula. B, The caustic holder. (From Bumstead Freeman J: The Pathology and Treatment of Venereal Diseases. Philadelphia, Blanchard and Lea, 1861.)*

was probably first accomplished by Dr. George Goodfellow about 1891.

At this point it becomes necessary to stray from history for a moment. Prostatectomy is usually the removal of prostatic adenomas, not the removal of the total prostate. Removal of the entire prostate with seminal vesicles is called radical prostatectomy. In prostatectomy, the adenomas are removed from the surgical capsule, which is formed of compressed normal prostatic tissues. Prostatic carcinoma, as well as recurrent adenomas, may still occur after prostatectomy. Radical prostatectomy leaves no remnant of the prostate and therefore no chance of prostatic carcinoma starting in tissues left behind. In 1904, Hugh Young, M.D., described several cases of radical perineal prostatectomy for carcinoma. None of his patients was cured, but all were improved. Young suggested the possibility of using this approach to cure prostatic cancer.

In the meantime, other approaches were being used to remove parts of the obstruction. Amussat removed what may have been a prostatic lobe in a suprapubic operation for stone in 1832. Prostatomes, or catheters and sounds carrying knife blades that could be concealed until utilized, became popular to cut the bladder neck and median bars. It must be understood that these were all blind operations, carried out with the aid of the tactile sense only.

The famous Leroy d'Étiolles thought a snare for intrusive prostatic lobes might give better hemostasis and he thought little of snaring a lobe and dragging it out through the

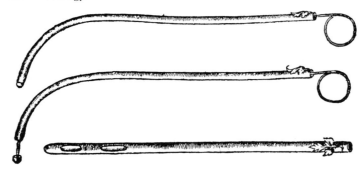

FIG. 44. *Pare's sounds with cutting edges for destroying carnosities. (From Pousson A, Desnos E (eds): Encyclopédie française d'urologie. Paris, Doin et Fils, 1914–1923.)*

urethra (Figs. 45 and 46). Various substances injected locally were also used in an attempt to shrink the obstructing glands. The necrosis, suppuration, and sepsis that often resulted soon stopped further attempts at this type of procedure. Freezing and dehydration used in modern times are direct descendants of this methodology, and results seem to differ little.

The first suprapubic approaches to the bladder were for the removal of stone or for the relief of urinary retention. When the retention was due to prostatic hypertrophy or bladder neck obstruction of any type, the cystotomy site would not close—a persistent fistulous tract remained to relieve the obstruction. If these eventually became strictured down, they were necessarily reopened. Prostatectomy through the suprapubic approach was described, advised, and written about by many, but it was not done with any facility or frequency until about 1890.

In 1878, C. W. Dulles of Philadelphia wrote:*

More than a hundred and fifty years ago, Cheselden, convinced by the demonstration of John Douglas that it was practicable to remove vesicle calculi by incision above the pubis, adopted this method, and carried it out so happily that he lost only one of ten patients, and

* Dulles, CW: *Am J Med Sci* 75:44–62, 1878.

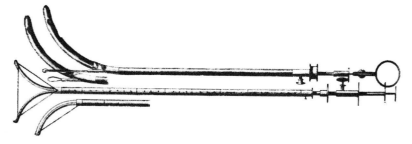

FIG. 45. *Prostatic cutting instrument, probably developed by Leroy d'Étiolles. (From Pousson A, Desnos E (eds) : Encyclopédie française d'urologie. Paris, Doin et Fils, 1914–1923.)*

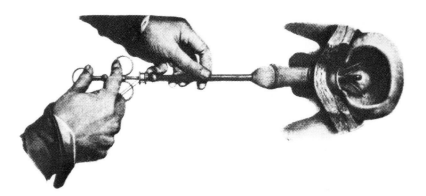

FIG. 46. *Leroy d'Étiolles' prostatic cutter—used to amputate a middle lobe of the prostate. (From Pousson A, Desnos E (eds): Encyclopédie française d'urologie. Paris, Doin et Fils, 1914–1923.)*

that one solely from his own extreme indiscretion. His great success, however, excited against him the jealousy and bitter animosity of Douglas, who persecuted him on account of his operation, accusing him of stealing credit which belonged right to another. At the same time, so rude was the surgery of that day, that other men, attempting this method, cut the peritoneum, and actually burst the bladder when they meant simply to distend it, which occurrences led Cheselden to leave off what he had so well begun, and go in search of some other way. This resulted in his applying his great skill to the perfecting of the method of Rau, converting it into that so universally known and practised [operation] as Cheselden's, or the lateral operation. Yet, for all this, he was not so much influenced by the sudden tide of alarm which had risen from the accidents alluded to, as to be blinded to the many advantages of the high or suprapubic operation. In giving his reasons for leaving it, he says: "Though this operation came into universal discredit, I must declare it my opinion that it is much better than the old way, to which they all returned, except myself, who would not have left the high operation, but for the hopes I had of a better, being well assured that it might hereafter be practised with greater success."

W. I. Belfield was one of the pioneers in the field of prostatic surgery. When surgical knowledge was far enough advanced to enable the use of sterile techniques, he attacked the prostate in two stages. The first step was to incise down to the bladder. Then, after a lapse of five to seven days, the bladder could be opened, surgical excision completed, and the bladder again closed. The first operations were removal of a lobe or lobes; this was soon followed by complete enucleations of the prostatic adenomas, usually accompanied by perineal drainage. Although Belfield was probably one of the first to plan this operation for the relief of prostatic obstruction and urinary retention, Leeds and von Dittell also resected prostatic portions suprapubically at about the same time.

In 1890, Belfield* reviewed all the published cases of prostatic surgery. He found 133 cases: one-third were operated perineally, two-thirds suprapubically, and four cases by both methods combined. Partial prostatectomy, severing of a median bar, and lobectomy were most often done, and about 68 percent of the patients were known to be able to have voluntary urination, postoperatively.

It is difficult for the modern surgeon to understand the hesitancy with which surgery was approached at the turn of

* Belfield, WI: Operation on the Enlarged Prostate, with a Tabulated Summary of Cases. *M J Med Sci* 100:439–452, 1890.

the century. There was at that time no awareness of the physiology of shock, sepsis, and uremia. There were no blood transfusions, blood expanders, antibacterials, or antibiotics. Morbidity and mortality were tremendously higher than one could now tolerate. Prostatic surgery was not approached until obstruction was total and the patient dangerously ill, and cure was accomplished when the patient could void, no matter how well.

I should like to quote Terence Millin, a fine gentleman who is known throughout the world for his development of the retropubic prostatectomy. While lecturing to our staff at Albert Einstein College of Medicine in 1970, he said:*

As far back as history records, man has been struggling to find a satisfactory way to deal with urinary obstruction due to the enlarged prostate gland. Early Chinese records and the tombs of the Egyptian pharaohs are said to have revealed evidence that various species of catheter were in use for this, but it was not until the closing years of the last century that a definitive operation became feasible, rendering it possible to establish a lasting cure—the removal of the whole of the hyperplastic glandular tissue.

The names of Belfield and Fuller in the United States and McGill in England were associated with the early suprapubic transvesical operations, which generally effected only a partial removal, and those of Proust in France and Young in the United States with the perineal operations. In 1901, Sir Peter Freyer, that controversial Irishman who practiced in London after a brief but lucrative career as an army surgeon in India, published his four cases of total prostatectomy, as he termed it. It seems certain that he got the idea from Ramon Guiteras of New York, who visited him at St. Peter's Hospital in London on his way to read a paper on the subject in Paris. It is probable, then, that Freyer does not deserve the widespread credit accorded to him for originality but he did lay down the main principles—complete removal of the hyperplastic tissue and adequate postoperative drainage, and his name was attached, certainly in Europe, to the procedure. It was, I think, Lord Moynihan who referred to this redoubtable protagonist as "that Galway man so aptly named 'pee-freer'."

* Herman John R: *Urology 1970.* Travenol Labs, Inc. Deerfield, Ill, 1970.

The next few decades saw dramatic changes in the surgery of the prostate, with introduction of satisfactory renal function tests, new drugs to combat sepsis, and the development of readily available blood transfusions; it is interesting to recollect that a mere forty years ago the three main causes of mortality were renal failure, urosepsis, and hemorrhage, with pulmonary complications not far behind. Today none of these is a real hazard, the main causes of death in the few who succumb from the operation being cardiovascular accidents and an occasional pulmonary embolus, and recent developments suggest that even these, or some of them, may yield to prompt therapeutic measures.

Although today few patients die as a result of prostatic surgery, we urologists must offer the patient more than just survival. He must have an improvement in his symptomatology, certainly not a worsening, and a warranty that his expectation of life will probably be lengthened. My own criteria for advising operation were pretty stringent. Broadly speaking, they fall under two headings: A, extreme symptomatology where we can offer relief and B, threatened renal deterioration due to back-pressure effects where operation is called for to save life. When acute retention has supervened, and one or more catheterizations have not reestablished micturition, intervention is also, of course, indicated. When symptoms of difficulty and urinary frequency are marked, the patient will seek relief. Here I would like to stress the necessity of proving actual obstruction, evidenced by bladder hypertrophy and trabeculation, in the case of the middle-aged man who presents himself with the sole symptom of urinary frequency, chiefly by day.

Eugene Fuller is accepted by most as the originator of the idea of suprapubic enucleation of the entire adenomatous prostate. Prior to that time the intravesical gland was cut out and the intraurethral gland attacked perineally. Fuller used his right hand to enucleate and with his left hand exerted perineal pressure to elevate the prostate within comfortable reach of his enucleating finger. Ramon Guiteras, a New York confrere of Fuller, inserted two fingers of his left hand into the rectum and used these fingers for pressure and guidance. Guiteras, on his way to the International Medical Congress in Paris, stopped off and met with Peter Freyer in Scotland. He is said to have described and even demonstrated the new operation, called by him "the rectovesical operation." Freyer then very promptly published his description of the procedure and claimed priority. Fuller refuted this, and there was considerable furor engendered by this published battle. The results were indefinite at the time, but the fight made the suprapubic approach popular and used by most surgeons of the time.

When I entered urology in 1927, the only prostate operation practised in Britain was the Freyer technique, usually handled as a two-stage procedure. Young's stout advocacy of the perineal approach went largely unheeded owing to the formidable and not infrequent complications encountered by those who assayed to follow the master. On the continent of Europe there were a few surgeons in Germany, Spain and Switzerland who utilized the approach but it was not popular. Indeed, it was said that in France no surgeon dared to employ it for fear of the common sequel of impotence, and people darkly hinted at the assassination of more than one urologist at the hands of a patient dissatisfied at such an outcome.

Until 1911, when J. Bentley Squier suggested opening the bladder high in the dome, it was usually opened just behind the pubis. The lower opening resulted in delayed closure. Squier's suggestion resulted in better and more rapid closures. When the operation was performed as a two-stage procedure, this was often done because of the dangers of catheter decompression of a long-standing obstruction. The acute decompression frequently resulted in uncontrollable hemorrhage; if that didn't end the patient's life, the sepsis that usually followed might. The two-stage procedure was therefore safer, because a catheter wasn't needed and a bladder opened widely and drained by incision was not as likely to bleed or develop sepsis. Von Zwallenburg and Bumpus were the two proponents of this new theory and proved that gradual decompression with a catheter could prevent hemorrhage and sepsis in the same way a cystostomy could.

Many other methods of prostatectomy were devised, and

many modifications of the original methods of Fuller and Guiteras were suggested. The hemostatic bag, the Marion tube, the Pilcher bag, the three-way Foley catheter, the starch cone, and the absorbable cellulose pack were all ways of controlling hemorrhage from the prostatic fossa. Suturing the bladder neck, packing with ribbed dam, and packing with gauze were all used for this same purpose. All were successful in the hands of some urologists; none were successful in the hands of all urologists. To date, different methods are still used in different clinics and in different parts of the world. Few close the bladder tightly without drainage, even now. The suggestion that a cystostomy Foley catheter be brought out through a stab wound separate from the incision has made it possible to expect the cystostomy fistula to be dry a few hours after removal of the catheter. In the old way, when the cystostomy Malecott, or "mushroom" catheter drainage was brought out through the incision, it sometimes required days or even weeks for the resulting fistula to close. Because the wound often became infected and broke down, secondary closures of suprapubic wounds were not infrequent.

TUR: The Development
of Instruments

Another popular method of prostatectomy is via the transure-thral route. When Hugh Young first produced his cold punch for removal of portions of the prostate, he started a progression of instruments that developed with little interruption to today's fine resectoscopes.

Young's punch consisted of a rather large–diameter sheath with a large fenestration on its convex surface (Fig. 47). This was passed into the bladder with an obturator, which was then removed. The fenestration was pressed down onto the prostate or median bar, and a cylinder with a sharp leading edge fitting closely into the sheath was then passed, cutting off the portion of prostate protruding through the fenestration. The entire operation was done more by feel than by visual control. This was followed by the punch with the rotating cutting edge, then the illuminated resectoscope, and very shortly by the electric resectoscope. The Kerwin rotating electric resecto-scope was developed to counteract the bleeding that follows the cold punch method. With Dr. T. J. Kerwin's instrument, the electric current could be used to coagulate blood in the

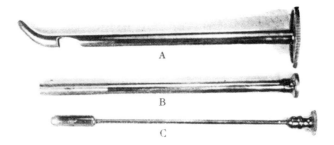

FIG. 47. *A. Outer sheath with fenestra, made of nonrusting steel. B. Inner cutting tube with inner portion of nonrusting steel. The outer portion is provided with notches to "connect with motor if desired." C. Obturator for introduction or removal of instrument.*

tissues before that portion of prostate was cut from its base. To do this, the tissue was pushed into the fenestration and a straight needle inserted in it. When the electric current had been used to coagulate vessels, the cutting blade was rotated, severing the coagulated tissues with minimal bleeding.

All these punch-type instruments were utilized with the theory that a bar or obstruction across the bladder neck could be cut, releasing the urine. There was little or no thought of resecting or removing the prostate, only making a channel.

Electrotherapy was probably first used about 1900; by 1909 Samuel-Jean Pozzi announced the cure of superficial and even of deep-seated cancers by high-frequency and high-tension sparks from the terminal of Paul Oudin's resonator, calling it "fulguration." This was a low-amperage current.

In New York, Dr. Finley Cook found the same effects serendipitously by short-circuiting a current to his finger and getting a burn. He treated skin tumors, warts, moles, and even infected tonsils and hemorrhoids.

Edwin Beer, a New York surgeon and urologist, first suggested and used high-frequency currents to destroy bladder tumors. In 1908, he applied the current through an early Nitze cystoscope. Howard A. Kelly in Baltimore took it up soon thereafter with his air cystoscopic speculum, and by 1914 it was in fairly widespread use in urologic circles over the world.

Probably the first urologic instrument used with the electric current was Enrico Bottini's galvanocautery: two closely aligned insulated brass arms passed as one instrument to produce thermogalvanic destruction of the prostate or bladder neck (Fig. 48). It was excellent in median-bar obstruction and caused few hemorrhages or sequelae. This was used blindly, but Albert Freudenberg invented an instrument using a similar cautery blade with a cystoscope so that the procedure could be controlled visually.

About 1890 to 1895, W. N. Wishard used a perineal approach and a modified rectal speculum to cauterize under direct observation.

C. H. Chetwood developed his own instrument for a perineal approach in about 1905. His operation was successful and used by many. The instrument rapidly went into disuse when suprapubic prostatectomy became the operation of choice.

Young started the cycle again when he showed how his punch could be used easily in a transurethral approach to median-bar and small bladder neck obstructions.

Beer's proof that the Oudin unipolar current could be used under water to cure bladder tumors resulted in his being awarded a gold medal, and in stimulating many urologists to use electricity. A. R. Stevens used a steel wire electrode in a catheterizing cystoscope to cauterize the offending prostatic lobes. He found that shrinkage sufficient to enable urination was obtainable with adequate use of the electrocurrent. No hemorrhage, no abdominal incision, and no need for hospitalization were the three main points favoring its use. H. G. Bugbee also used the Oudin current; he found he could destroy the median bar and burn a channel between the lateral lobes adequate for urination. Following this, others began to use electric methods to produce a tunnel for urination.

Georges Luys, in France, suggested his "forage de la prostate," during which, over a period of weeks or months in

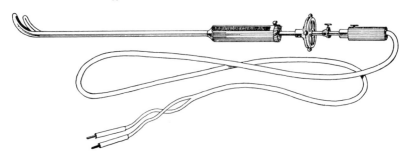

FIG. 48. *Bottini's galvanocautery. (From Deaver John B: Enlargement of the Prostate. Blakiston, 1905.)*

repeated operations, a channel is burned for passage of urine.

William F. Braasch modified Young's punch so that it could be controlled visually and very shortly thereafter Young supplanted the cylindric cutting sheath with a tubular cautery. This didn't become popular because it didn't work easily and it grounded out too often. John R. Caulk, also of the United States, constructed an electropunch that worked somewhat better but was still unsatisfactory. Several others made attempts, more or less successful, at electrifying Young's punch. K. M. Walker, A Londoner, first suggested the Bakelite, or nonconductive, sheath for this instrument.

The first major new step came in 1926, when Dr. Maximilian Stern of New York devised a tungsten loop that was movable and could cut cylinders of tissue from the tissue that could be pushed into the fenestration. Telescopes could be used to locate and position the fenestra properly, and then another telescope was used to direct this cutting loop in its excursions.

Herman Bumpus suggested the use of the Bugbee electrode for control of bleeding after resection and he remarked there could be no contraindications to reoperation if the obstruction grew back.

Reinhold Wappler worked on the problem of the undependable electric currents, and developed the radiotherm about 1922 or 1923. Urologists were not impressed by its reliability; shortly thereafter a spark-gap cutting machine, the electrotome, was produced. This current cut as well under water as in air and with little or no coagulation of tissues. Wappler modified the panendoscope system to utilize the foroblique lens with the electrified blade. Hemorrhage was still a problem, and T. M. Davis now combined the cutting current with a diathermy machine for hemostasis, achieving commendable results. He also used a heavier tungsten wire loop, which proved much less friable. During the operations with this equipment, a double-throw foot switch was used to enable cutting or coagulation current to flow to the working element.

Joseph McCarthy, using this technique, worked with Wappler to develop an open-ended sheath of Bakelite. With this it was possible to survey the excursions of the loop and, cutting from inside the bladder toward the surgeon, delineate exactly the length of the segment of tissue removed and even the depth. This instrument, with modifications, is what most resectionists use today. When first introduced, it was used to resect several segments of an obstructing bar or lobe. It was not unusual in those days for an operative report to read: "3 segments removed," "5 pieces burned out," or "adequate channel made." TURP (transurethral resection of the prostate) meant exactly that; the prostatic obstruction was resected, not extirpated.

Foley invented an instrument with an electrified wire strung from the curved tip to the shaft. This wire bow could be revolved to cut a funnel of prostate, leading to removal of the entire prostate. The large pieces cut out then were cut into smaller segments for removal.

In almost all subsequent development of the resectoscope, the interest and abilities of Wappler were a very important factor. Kerwin developed a derivative of the punch instrument with a rotating wire electrode maintained within the fenestration of the sheath. This rotary resectoscope was presented in 1932.

The Stern–McCarthy resectoscope put the traveling loop on a rack and pinion handle to more precisely control its excursions. However, two hands were needed to operate this instrument. Reed M. Nesbit, thinking that no more than one hand should be used to operate it, placed an internal spring in the handle that would pull the loop into the sheath. The other hand was inserted into the rectum to stabilize the prostate. By this time Nesbit was doing a complete transurethral prostatectomy (TUP), no longer just a resection.

Baumrucker altered Nesbit's method by reversing the spring so that cutting was done against the spring "for better control." The accidents that resulted when unguarded relaxation caused the spring to extend the "hot" loop into the bladder, and perhaps through the bladder, militated against its popularity. Iglesias replaced the sometimes sticky internal coiled spring of Nesbit with an always reliable external leaf spring. In addition, the operating portion was made to accept different loop sizes and fit into woven silk or plastic sheaths of different sizes. This instrument is widely used today.

Frederick Wappler, Reinhold Wappler's son, was the chief originator of the vacuum tube oscillator, which delivered continuous or undamped electric oscillations of high frequency. This was a stable, controllable current, ideal for the urologist.

Transurethral electrosurgical prostatectomy has found favor in urologic services, and today no resident training program can be considered complete that does not teach these techniques.

Fiber optics probably developed as a result of efforts to make a flexible endoscope for examination of the stomach. As early as 1930 quartz fibers had been tried for this purpose unsuccessfully. Glass fibers, when bundled, failed to give clear light transmission, because the light was not maintained in each fiber: it deteriorated in quantity and quality as it voyaged from one fiber to another. The next efforts were to make a glass fiber with a high refractive index in an attempt to maintain the light within the fiber and so prevent the losses by "contamination." This type of fiber transmitted about one-third of the light passed into it. When these fibers were loosely grouped, the image was good—that is, sharp. However, when the fibers were bundled firmly together, as required for an instrument, the image became blurred and washed out. This was due again to leakage from fiber to fiber because of irregularities at the interfaces.

In 1956, Lawrence E. Curtiss made glass fibers from highly refractive glass rod within glass tubing of low refractive index. This was a non-scattering, controlled, virtually indestructible fiber without interface losses. A bundle of these fibers three feet long was the basis of the first gastroscope that was fully flexible. It was first used at the University of Michigan in 1957. In 1958, the three who had done most of the early work on fiber optics—Curtiss, Basil I. Hirschowitz, and C. Wilbur Peters—became associated with American Cystoscope Makers, Inc. Their purpose was to further develop the technology and mechanics of fiber optics used in gastroscopes and other endoscopes, including cystoscopes. The gastroduodenal fiberscope was the first production model of a fiber optic instrument. The fiber optic cystoscope was soon in production and is rapidly replacing the incandescent bulb scope.

Aphrodisiacs

No history of urology would be complete without some discussion of aphrodisiacs. Aphrodisiacs have been of two basic types: those intended to cause someone else to fall in love with a person, and those thought to give an individual more desire for sexual contacts and more capability for sexual acts. The first type of love powders and potions is well-illustrated in Shakespeare's *A Midsummer Night's Dream,* in which Titania is given a love philter on her eyelids as she sleeps. On awakening she falls in love with the first person she sees; this happens to be Bottom, who has the head of an ass. This type of potion, interesting as it is, will not be the topic of our discussion. We shall dwell only on those therapeutics designed to increase the sexual abilities and desires of men and women.

To quote John Davenport:*

When it is considered how strongly the sexual desire is implanted in man, and how much his self-love is interested in preserving or in recovering the power of gratifying it, his endeavors to infuse fresh vigour into his organs when they are temporarily exhausted by over-indulgence or debilitated by age cannot appear surprising.

* Davenport John: *Aphrodisiacs and Anti-Aphrodisiacs.* London, Privately printed, 1869.

This remark particularly applies to natives of southern and eastern climes, with whom the erotic ardour makes itself more intensely felt; since it is there that man's imagination, as burning as the sky beneath which he first drew breath, reawakens desires his organs may long have lost the power of satisfying, and consequently it is there more especially that, not withstanding the continual disappointment of his hopes, he still pertinaciously persists in searching for means whereby to stimulate his appetite for sexual delights. Accordingly it will be found that even in the remotest ages, the animal, vegetable, and mineral kingdoms have been ransacked for the purpose of discovering remedies capable of strengthening the genital apparatus and exciting it to action.

But however eager men might be in the above enquiry, their helpmates were equally desirous of finding a means whereby they might escape the reproach of barrenness—a reproach than which none was more dreaded by eastern women.

Mandrake (*Mandragora officinarum*) is a plant with a carrot-like root, usually divided from the middle downward, having roughly the shape of the lower parts of the human body. This was mentioned for its enhancement of fertility in the Bible (Genesis 30:14–17), and by Pythagoras, Plutarch, and many others. Belief in its value as a love philter, or love potion, and as an aid to fertility in barren women was widespread; in some areas, it is still sold for that purpose. It is used to "excite the amorous propensity, remedy female sterility, facilitating conception and prolificness." There is also the interesting fable that ". . . female elephants, after eating its leaves, are seized with so irresistible a desire for copulation, as to run eagerly, in every direction, in quest of the male."

"Man-like" was the name given by Pythagoras, "semihomo" by Columella, and "mandragora" by others. Rudely carved figurines were sold at fairs and markets. Machiavelli wrote a play about "La Mandragora" in the fifteenth century. Mandrake was mentioned by many authors through the years; even now in many countries mandrake root is available in the marketplace. Mandrake, however, was mostly famed for its connection with fertility. Years before its mention, other drugs were used to increase sexual potency.

Since the first penis was found to be soft when it should have been hard, man has known the suffering associated with impotence. Since those first times centuries ago, man has sought remedies for this condition, almost always looking outside himself rather than within his mind and body. The famous Hindu *Vedas*—heroic poems handed down for generations from father to son—discussed these situations in full, without skirting the condition in any way. The *Sushruta Samhita,* probably originating more than 3000 years ago, contains an entire section devoted to the Vaji-Karana (aphrodisiac) remedies:*

If duly taken, the Vaji-Karana remedies make a man sexually as strong as a horse [Vaji] and enable him cheerfully to satisfy the heat and amorous ardours of young maidens, a fact which has determined the nomenclature of this class of remedies . . . that which creates spontaneous pleasurable excitement, the therapy which bestows considerable sexual stamina and by the use of which therapy a person is most liked by members of the opposite sex.

Various kinds of nutritious and palatable food and sweet, luscious and refreshing liquid cordials, speech that gladdens the ears, and touch which seems delicious to the skin, clear nights mellowed by the beams of the full moon and damsels young, beautiful and gay; dulcet songs that charm the soul and captivate the mind, use of Betal-leaves, wine, wreaths of sweet scented flowers and a merry careless heart—these are the best aphrodisiacs of life.

A youth in sound health taking regularly some sort of Vaji-Karana remedy may enjoy the pleasures of youth every night during all seasons of the year. Old men, those wishing to enjoy sexual pleasures or to secure the affections of women, as well as those suffering from senile decay or sexual incapacity, and persons weakened from sexual excesses should do well to submit themselves to a course of Vaji-Karana remedies. They are highly beneficial to gay, handsome, and opulent youths and to persons who have many wives.

The very interesting and at times introspective *Sushruta Samhita* goes into the causes of impotence and describes six

* Bhishagratna KL: *An English Translation of the Sushruta Samhita.* Varanasi, India; Chowkhamba Sanskrit Series Office, 1963.

types—voluntary, congenital, praecox, those due to diseases of the genitals and so on. Mental impotence is described and a sample case given:

A cessation of the sexual desire owing to the rising of the bitter thoughts of recollection on the mind of a man, or a forced intercourse with a disagreeable woman (one who fails sufficiently to rouse up the sexual desire in the heart of her mate), illustrates an instance of mental impotency.

Some of the remedies and their very interesting results are described:

Utkaria—powders of sesame, Masha pulse, and S'ali rice should be mixed with Saindhava salt and mashed with sugar cane. This then is mixed with hog's lard and cooked with clarified butter. By using this Utkaria a man would be able to visit a hundred women.

By eating the testes of a he–goat with an adequate quantity of salt and powdered pepper fried in a clarified butter prepared from churning milk (and not from curd), a man is enabled to visit a hundred women one after the other.

Powdered pipal, pepper, Masha pulse, rice, wheat and barley in equal parts are made into cakes and fried in clarified butter. By taking these cakes and a potion of milk sweetened with a copious quantity of sugar, a man becomes potent enough to enjoy the pleasures of love like a sparrow.

Powdered vidari soaked in juice of same and dried and coated with honey in clarified butter . . . whereby a man would be able to visit ten women successively.

Powders of dried amalaka successively soaked in its own expressed juice, licked or coated with honey, sugar and clarified butter, after which a quantity of milk should be taken. This compound makes even an old man of eighty sexually as vigorous as a youth.

One very interesting remedy described is especially so because of its mode of attack and results:

Clarified butter should be boiled with eggs or testes of alligators, mice, frogs, and sparrows. By lubricating the sole of the feet with this, a man would be able to visit a woman with undiminished vigour as long as he would not touch the ground with his feet.

Another remedy guaranteed to increase semen quantity and quality and also increase the libido, if all the ingredients were pure and without adulteration. Still another remedy made of large amounts of pepper plus other material promised that "he who drinks this, according to the strength of his gastric fire, will not suffer phallic depression or ejaculation for the whole night."

The problems of impotence have been discussed in writing from almost all civilizations. The *Nei-Ching* discusses the philosophy of impotence. The *Aqrābādhīn of Al-Kindī,* an Arabian text, gives prescriptions for oil of jasmine and asafetida, as does the *Sushruta Samhita:*

Throw in good oil of jasmine and asafetida and leave it for some days. Then the male organ is oiled with that oil of jasmine at the time of intercourse. The woman is excited by its contact and she experiences a strong lust. This causes pregnancy. The woman who is not excited for intercourse and has not the inclination of it is treated with this.

Hippocrates, discussing the Scythian, is quoted as having said:

In addition, there are many eunuchs amongst the Scythians who perform female work and speak like women. Such persons are called effeminates. The inhabitants of this country attribute the cause of their impotence to a god, and venerate and worship such persons, everyone dreading that the like may befall himself. To me it appears that such affectations are just as much divine as all others are, and that no one disease is either more divine or more human than another—and that no one arises without a natural cause.

But these complaints befell the Scythians, and they are the most impotent of men—because they always wear breeches and spend most of their time on horseback, so as not to touch their privy parts with the hand, and from the cold and fatigue they forget the sexual desire, and do not make the attempt until after they have lost their virility.

Coming to a more modern time, Edward Martin in 1895 wrote:* "The treatment of psychical impotence will be successful in its issue in accordance with the power of the physician to make upon the mind of this patient a strong impression."

Mankind had traveled through the age of gods and witchcraft into modernity, but as Henry Sigerist very wisely said:* "Impotence, however, like other nervous disorders and particularly sexual neurosis, is still a playground of superstition and quackery."

In 1940, Wilhelm Stekel found impotence to be a disorder of modern civilization:* "The majority of civilized men have neither the time nor the energy for love."

In the early 1900s, Serge Voronoff, Director of the Laboratory of Experimental Surgery of the College of France, began publishing his results with monkey glands. His works were numerous and published in several countries. He wrote of ovarian grafts, thyroid gland grafts, skin grafts, bone grafts, and other types of experimental surgery. His name and fame, however, came as a result of his claim of rejuvenation by grafting ape glands to men. Two titles are significant: *The Study of Old Age and My Method of Rejuvenation* and *The Conquest of Life* were probably on the best–seller lists of some aphrodisiac clubs. To quote the author: "This method, as applied to a large number of human subjects, has yielded positive results, both physical and mental, not only to ourselves but to our faithful collaborators Dartigues and Georges Voronoff, who have performed hundreds of grafting operations, and also to a number of others."

* Herman John R: Impotencia Throughout the Ages. *J Am Soc Psychosom Dent Med* 16:93–99, 1969.

Voronoff used the ape as a donor:*

. . . an animal possessing the closest zoological similarity with man, the anthropoid ape, which most nearly approaches the human species in the highly perfected development of its tissues and in its intimate humoral chemism. . . . the graft employed is really not a heterograft, but a graft between two closely related species, such as may be made between the dog and wolf, or between the rabbit and the hare. The graft employed between species so closely related as this is very far from the heterograft, and, on the other hand, is closely related to the homograft. It may be termed, "homeo-graft," the organs of one species finding identical conditions of life on the organism of a nearly allied species.

Voronoff made four grafts from one testicle, quartering it and then placing it on the tunica vaginalis because of its rich blood supply. His description of the amazing results may also be of interest:

In the majority of cases, marked psychical and sexual excitation occurs in man during the first few days following testicular transplantation. The patients believe that this abrupt phenomenon is a sign of the beneficial effects of the procedure. However, these results continue only for a few days and the supposed good effects rapidly diminish and usually completely disappear. For the first two months, and often during the first three months, after grafting the patient experiences no beneficial effect whatever, at least so far as objective evidence is concerned. This period is one of disappointment, disillusion and discouragement and commonly follows the enthusiasm present during the immediately early period.

However, the satisfaction and pleasure of the patient become so much the greater, later on. In the course of two or three months, marked improvement in the psychic functions occurs, especially in physicians and other individuals who are highly developed intellectually. There are improvements in memory, greater aptitudes for mental labour and greater facility for intellectual effort. At the same time the genital functions become more active and a general condi-

* Voronoff Serge, Alexandrescu George: *Testicular Grafting from Ape to Man.* Translated by Theodore C Merrill, MD, Brentano, Ltd., circa 1930.

tion and sensation of well being occurs. Such are the earlier phenomena observed.

Other improvements noted: disappearance of wrinkles, increase in body hair, brighter eyes, invigoration of the enfeebled body, decrease in subcutaneous fat, increase in appetite, blood pressure decrease in hypertensives, improved urinary evacuation, and so on. The effects of the graft begin to diminish and completely disappear after the fifth or sixth year. Voronoff's works span almost 25 years, nearly up to 1930, during which hundreds of grafts were sold, and controversy in the medical profession raged.

Goat glands became popular shortly thereafter in the southwestern United States and a tremendous business empire was built on this improbability.

One of the blue bloods of the Caribbean was asked to what he owed his manliness. In an offhand manner, he is said to have reported that he drank rum in which pago palo had been soaked. This material, the bark and roots of a tree found in the Caribbean, became a much sought after commodity and the price soared.

In New York, San Francisco, Tokyo, Paris, and other great cities of the world, there are currently sex stores, nature stores, and pharmacies that sell and specialize in aphrodisiacs. The rhinoceros in Africa has become an endangered species because of the demand for rhinoceros horn as an aphrodisiac. Oysters have been jokingly referred to as a food for "lovers" over the years, and yet there have been no proven aphrodisiacs up until these last few years. One of the side effects of L-dopa is that it sometimes acts as an aphrodisiac to a very small percentage of males taking it for Parkinson's disease. This fact has served as stimulus for several research projects!

Bladder Tumors

One of the lesser known facets of the history of urology is that relating to bladder tumors. At present we insert a cystoscope, see the tumor, biopsy it, and decide which approach we think is best suited to that individually placed, histologically diagnosed, and staged lesion.

'Twas not always so. Hippocrates may or may not have known of bladder tumors when in his aphorisms he stated: "Blood or pus in the urine indicated ulceration either of the kidney or the bladder," and that where ". . . furfuraceaous particles discharged along with thick urine, there is scabies of the bladder." He at least knew of bladder-neck obstructions and probably of tumors as well. We have no records of the Egyptians or Hindus recognizing this separate entity, but some of their records could be translated to indicate bladder neoplasms.

The first actual record we have referring to bladder tumors directly is probably from a monograph by Lacuna, published in Rome in 1551. In it, Lacuna recognizes and describes carnosities of the bladder and caruncles of the bladder neck.

Pierre Franco is said to have made a suprapubic incision to remove a lesion that he found he could not remove from the bladder in the more usual perineal approach. There must have been many calcium-encrusted, large tumors that were mistaken for vesical calculi and operated on by the lithotomists. Perhaps these were the soft stones sometimes remarked.

Joseph Covillard of France, in 1639, in a monograph entitled *Surgical Observations on Curious and Unique Cases* [the translation is mine, from *Observations intra chirurgiques pleines des remarques curieuses et evenements singuliers*] reported on a deliberate perineal approach to the bladder for removal of neoplasm. J. Warner* reported that he incised the urethra of a woman, drew out a bladder tumor, and tied off the pedicle with complete cure. Such courage caused others to follow this lead.

Many reports then began to appear and discussions were noted about the benign bladder fungus or carnosities now known as papillomas and cancerous tumors; many different and ingenious means were used to attempt to cure these lesions. François Chopart in his *Treatment of Illness of the Urinary Passages* [*Traité des maladies des voies urinaires*], published in France in 1791, distinguishes between bladder tumors and tumors of the neck of the bladder. He emphasized that urinary bleeding might well be due to tumors and thought that benign fungoid tumors could become cancerous.

Many were the ingenious attempts to remove and cure these lesions. The well-known physicians of the time each had his own method. Jean Civiale attempted to grasp and tear them out; Leroy d'Étiolles attempted to crush the base and pull them out. Looping, scraping, squeezing, and tieing off were all methods used for this purpose. Most of the knowledge of these lesions was obtained at autopsy.

Theodor Bilroth, the famous German surgeon, opened the modern era of bladder tumor surgery about 1874, when he published a case describing the suprapubic approach (Franco did it almost three hundred years earlier) and removal of a large bladder tumor from a child. An excellent surgeon, well-

* Warner J: *Cases in Surgery*. 1781.

based in anatomic knowledge, he opened the bladder widely and under direct vision removed the tumor. Trendelenburg, Volkmann, Dittel, Guyon, and Albarran—all famous surgeons with worldwide reputations—began using the suprapubic approach for bladder surgery. Others continued with the perineal approach in spite of this.

Eduard Sonnenburg may well have been the first to attempt to remove a part of the bladder wall with the tumor. His patient's lesion must have been in the posterior dome of the bladder, because he removed the bladder wall and also the covering peritoneum. The patient died within the month. Shortly after this, the modern method of extraperitonealization of the bladder was described. This made resections of the bladder wall much more feasible and, of course, more popular.

Three means of getting at these bladder lesions were in use: suprapubic, perineal, and transurethral. The perineal approach was soon given up when it became obvious that, with the aid of the cystoscope, inspection of the entire interior of the bladder was available and, in the Trendelenburg position, the entire bladder could be reached surgically. It was all due to the great advances of the cystoscope and its newer adaptations to biopsy instruments that this became possible.

Max Nitze operated cystocopically on bladder tumors in more than one hundred and fifty cases. He used a snare and a cautery, first cutting off the tumor and then burning its base. Nitze was specific and advised this only for the benign lesions, and he was able to cure a number of his patients who had benign papillomas. Nitze may well have been the first to differentiate bladder tumors into benign and malignant, replacing the previously held belief that all bladder tumors were malignant, just more or less so. Not all were able to duplicate Nitze's methods, however. Nitze's instrument was bulky, mechanically inefficient by today's standards, and hard to use by any standards. Other methods to destroy tumors were badly needed.

Edwin Beer, urologist and surgeon, showed that the Oudin current utilized through heavily insulated electrodes could be used with the cystoscope to destroy tumors. He consulted with Reinhold Wappler, who made the Oudin apparatus. Wappler advised against its use with a cystoscope, fearing the current would burn out the cystoscope and believing also that an air gap was needed between the applicator and the tumor. Beer experimented with the current, led through a cystoscope, to burn warts off a hand held in water. This worked, and in 1910 Beer destroyed in "several short settings" two tumors in elderly women.

Wappler in the meantime, apparently intrigued with this problem, suggested to E. L. Keyes that a bipolar current be used to burn tumors. He required two electrodes at first, one on each side of the lesion; but he soon found that one electrode could be placed under the patient's hips or back, and only one active electrode was needed on the lesion. The Jacques d'Arsonval (bipolar) current rapidly replaced the Oudin (monopolar) type. The simplicity of its application and its readily available equipment have caused its rapid adoption throughout the urologic and surgical world.

Forceps manufactured by Wappler for the Buerger cystoscope, rongeurs invented by Hugh H. Young, and other instruments were all used to obtain biopsies of the growth and to speed up its removal cystoscopically.

Others suggested intravesical instillations of escharotics— chemicals used to destroy the neoplasms. This complicated and dangerous method proved unsatisfactory, as did the use of intravesical radium salts, which was the first step in a new development featuring tumor irradiation.

R. Paschkis tried radium salts in 1911. Young tried radium with electrocautery fulguration and diathermy, but it was too complicated and time consuming. Thus, when B. S. Barringer and Abraham Hyman found they could use radium emanations, the popularity of this method was assured. Glass seeds, then gold seeds, containing radium emanations and called radon seeds, were used. These were implanted in geometric patterns, by means of flexible elongated needles, through the scope. First the seed was placed in the needle and held there by a touch of Vaseline. The needle was then passed through the scope and into the base of the lesion; the plunger was injected and the seed ejected into the tissues. Experts in this method would make a carefully calculated pattern of seeds that by x ray would seem almost exact. Memorial Hospital and Mt. Sinai Hospital in New York City were among the earliest to use and popularize this method of therapy.

In the meantime, surgical therapy was progressing also. Total removal of tumor without removal of the bladder wall resulted in recurrences so often that bladder wall resection was often attempted. Total cystectomy—probably first done in Germany by Bernhard Bardenheuer in 1887—was suggested also.

Edwin Beer demonstrated his surgical method in the early 1900s, and he proved that the extraperitoneal approach was much safer, with lower mortality and morbidity. It also enabled resection of the trigonal area and reimplantation of the ureter, if needed. Use of the bipolar current suprapubically to coagulate completely the portion of tumor that could be seen was used in an attempt to prevent implantation of the lesion due to surgery during partial resections.

Beer also advised total cystectomy in cases of malignant tumors—he transplanted the ureters to the skin. Robert C. Coffey placed the ureters into the sigmoid. The use of the ileal loop was to come along fifty years later. Statistical studies of therapy with radical surgical approaches were made by the group at Memorial Hospital headed by Marshall and Whitemore. They did cystectomy, radical cystectomy with pelvic dissection, pelvic exenteration, and dissection up to the renal arteries. Their results stressed the importance of histologic grading and anatomic staging. The grading is the attempt to classify the lesion according to its malignancy, and it is done on the basis of cellular differentiation, mitotic figures, and so on. Staging is the attempt to show how far the lesion had spread when it is removed. Grading and staging proved valuable in estimating prognosis, but unfortunately, when based on biopsy they *only* reveal the characteristics of that portion of tissue removed. True classification remained to be established after removal of the entire lesion. This is perhaps straying from history a bit, but to understand some of the historic papers regarding bladder tumors, these facts must be made clear.

New methods were also being developed in external radiation therapy with deep radiation. The value of this in bladder tumors is still being argued because staging and grading cannot be considered accurate when the lesion cannot be removed and examined.

The transurethral approach received a big boost when resectoscopes were developed to the point where the Stern–McCarthy instrument was available. This made bladder tumors available to all urologists endoscopically. The further development of instruments for transurethral treatment of bladder lesions has been spelled out in detail in Chapter 12.

Urinalysis

Although examination of the urine by uroscopists and doctors was noted in the earliest records, modern urinary examinations began only when doctors stopped looking through urine and began looking into it.

Egyptians recorded hematuria, incontinence of urine, and burning of the urine. They also used human and animal urines for medication. Lest we react in horror and surprise to this early use of urine, be aware that in a book published in 1944, John W. Armstrong described "urine-therapy."* His *Water of Life* describes fasting and drinking one's own urine for healing, rebuilding, and reconditioning the body. And he was not alone in advising this therapy.

Aetius of Mesopotamia wrote an entire book on uroscopy in 500 AD and by 1130 AD Actuarius found the relation between exposure to cold and hemoglobinuria. Ten years later *Liber de Urinus,* a book classifying diseases solely on the basis of urinary changes, was released.

Urine samples classically were gathered in a matula for

* Armstrong John W: *Water of Life.* London, True Health Publishing Co., 1944.

examination. This bulbous clear glass container was divided into four parts corresponding to the head, breast, stomach, and urinary organs. The changes seen in these parts of the matula identified the location and the nature of the malady.

Fletcher,* writing about the time Vesalius described renal anatomy, told of the differences, causes, and judgments of urine. He suggested checking the whole urine, "but mingle not the urines that are made at separate times, but keep them separate both for quantity, color, and contents." In other words he advised "fractional" urine examinations. He classified 15 different colors of urine.

When uroscopy was at its peak, there were few other diagnostic or clinical testing methods known. Inspection of the urine became more popular and more spectacular, and more of an art than a science. It was done by doctors, uroscopists, watercasters, and even traveling water doctors. These travelers had a good thing going. They would load up with glass matulas and set up a stand in a new village. Customers could take a matula home in its wicker basket and then bring it back filled. The traveling man would examine and diagnose, and prescribe medication that he would then sell. Next day or so, he moved on to new territory before any results of his diagnosis and therapy became known.

Paracelsus believed people were composed of mercury, sulfur, and salt; proper treatment could result from learning which of these were in inappropriate quantities in the urine, which he distilled for his tests.

In 1620, uric acid's rhomboidal bricks, or crystals, were described; at about the same time, the specific gravity of the urine was given as the main diagnostic guide to illnesses. The early Egyptian findings of honey urine were repeated as a new discovery about 1675 by Thomas Willis. He found sweet urine in diabetics. By the mid-eighteenth century, Lorenzo Bellini was evaporating urines and Hermann Boerhaave was measuring the quantity and specific gravity of urine. Boerhaave

---

* Fletcher: *The Differences, Causes and Judgments of Urine Analysis.* Lecture Memoranda AMA, London, Burroughs Wellcome & Co., 1911.

recognized that any substance existing in the urine was derived from the blood.

Urea was extracted at this same time, and Matthew Dobson boiled diabetic's urine and derived a white crystalline cake indistinguishable from sugar by taste or smell. William Cruickshank probably discovered a chemical test for albumin when he added nitrous acid to urine from a patient with "dropsy" and got a precipitate.

Litmus papers were used in urine in the early 1800s, and albumin was described and tested for at the same time. However, urinalysis in relation to illness and therapy was not widely used until after the work of Richard Bright, physician and pathologist. In 1827, he wrote of dropsy and hydropic patients, and the results of his postmortum findings: *

I have never yet examined the body of a patient dying with dropsy, attended with coaguable urine, in which some obvious derangement was not discovered in the kidneys. In all the cases which I have observed the albuminous urine, it has appeared to me that the kidney has itself acted a more important part and has been more deranged both functionally and organically than has generally been imagined.

He summarized one of his autopsy reports: "In this case, again, we distinctly trace the existence of a highly diseased condition of the kidney coupled with the secretion of albuminous urine." Bright was the first scientist to connect a finding in the urine with a clinical disease entity. Kidney disease for a time became known as Bright's disease. This work marked the turning point. After Bright's time, urinalysis was conducted on a scientific basis.

Casts were soon described by Golding Bird, who made an atlas of findings in the urine sediment. Uric acid and urea were tested for quantitatively, and in 1847 Marwick wrote a

* Bright Richard: *Report of Medical Cases Selected With a View of Illustrating The Symptoms and Cure of Disease by a reference to Morbid Anatomy*. Vol I, London, 1827.

guide to scientific urinalysis including litmus, specific gravity, and albumin and sugar tests by copper reduction.

Urinalysis soon became widely accepted by physicians as an aid to clinical diagnosis and therapy. It became a truly monstrous procedure, requiring hours and resulting in chemical analysis so detailed as to be practically useless for active practice. The pendulum had swung too far. Bird suggested limiting the examination to isolation of those ingredients of recognized pathologic importance. Urophain, uroxanthum, hippuric acid, creatinin, fat, sulfides, carbonate of ammonia, sulfuret of ammonia, ammonium magnesium phosphates, bile pigment, carbonate of soda, lead, silver, gold, and others were all on the usual list of materials routinely tested for at that time, as were inosite, cystin, tyrosin, leucin, and other materials.

Henry Bence-Jones wrote about the protein that bears his name:*

On the first of November 1845, I received from Dr. Watson the following note with a test tube containing a thick yellow semisolid substance. "The tube contains urine with a very high specific gravity; when boiled it becomes highly opaque; on the addition of nitric acid it effervesces, assumes a reddish hue, becomes quite clear, but, as it cools, assumes the consistence and appearance which you see: heat reliquifies it. What is it?" His conclusion after study: "It is an oxide of albumin, and from the ultimate analysis, it is the hydrated deutoxide of albumin. This was in a case of "mollities ossium." . . . This substance must be looked for in acute cases of mollities ossium.

Shortly thereafter, John Charles Weaver Lever found albumin in the urine of eclamptic women and his may have been the first application of knowledge of albumin to obstetric practice. He did urine studies on all obstetric patients at Guys Hospital and discovered albumin only in women who had convulsions or "precursors to puerperal fits."

---

* Bence-Jones Henry: A New Substance Occurring in the Urine of a Patient with Mollitis Ossium. *Philosophical Transactions* 2:673, 1850.

These were important times for the development of urinalysis. In 1857, acetone was described in the urine of diabetics by Wilhelm Petters, and in 1861 Bödeker found alcaptones. Lead, inosite, and nitrites were found, and tests were derived for their determinations. Pyknometers were devised for specific-gravity testing, and Peter A. Griess, a German chemist, developed a reagent for the detection of nitrite in solutions by forming red azo dyes. This test, of little importance to urinalysis by itself, was to be used for the basis of the first dipsticks widely used as the Stat test in 1966.

In 1870, Austin Flint, Jr., published his *Manual of Chemical Examination of the Urine in Disease.** This book soon became a classic and sold through many editions. His main aim ". . . has been to enable the busy practitioner to make for himself, rapidly and easily, all ordinary examination of urine." He set up standards for instruments and testing equipment (Figs. 49 and 50). He said: "It is now so easy to make examinations of the urine extended and accurate enough for ordinary clinical purposes, that there is no good reason why physicians, especially recent graduates, should not be able to ascertain for themselves most of the important facts to be learned from a urinary analysis, and this without an undue expenditure of time and pains."

The colorimetric determinations of urea in urine by Otto Folin and H. Wu came to change much of the chemical analysis of urine in 1919; Francis Benedict in 1922 developed a direct determination of uric acid. Soon the pendulum was to swing away from the popularity and importance of urinalysis toward the importance of blood tests.

Edward Keyes, a prominent urologist, commented in 1928 on the striking difference between urinalysis as practiced by a urologist on a fresh specimen with his own microscope, and that by an internist who sends it to a laboratory.

---

* Flint Austin, Jr: *Manual of Chemical Examination of the Urine in Disease.* New York, D Appleton & Co., 1870.

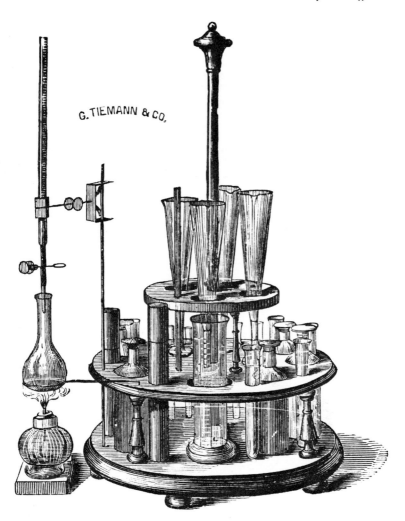

FIG. 49. *Laboratory set up for urinalysis. (From Catalogue of G Tiemann & Co, 1879.)*

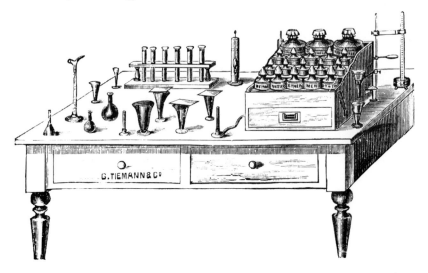

FIG. 50. *Work bench set up for the laboratory testing of urines. (From Catalogue of G Tiemann & Co, 1879.)*

The electrophoretic tests, the Addis counts, and the Papanicolaou tests all came before 1950. The Ames Company came out with the first dipsticks called Clinistix soon thereafter; at present, the microscope, dipsticks, and urinometer are all that are needed for most clinical urine examinations.

Odds and Ends

Odd ideas and dead ends, that is. The history of urology, as almost any other history of progress, is filled with peculiar ideas that became popular fads in urologic circles, or became dead ends developmentally.

For instance, floating kidney or nephroptosis was considered a very important entity in the early 1900s. Roentgenograms revealed the kidney one, two, or three vertebral spaces lower when the patient was upright than when he was prone. The kinking of the ureter was shown and was thought to explain the pain in these patients. By surgically fixing the kidney up under the ribs, either to the periostium or rib itself, there was no ptosis and no kinking and so no obstruction. Lucky patients were told to wear a corset, put on weight, or whatever, in an attempt to prove or disprove that nephroptosis was the cause of severe colic. Some diagnosticians pontificated that if a good, solid girdle prevented recurrence of back pain when worn over a long period (Fig. 51), then nephropexy or nephrorrhaphy was certainly indicated. Joseph Dietl described the crisis he thought occurred because of acute arterial kinking when the kidney dropped. Dietl's crisis was diagnosed frequently. In 1914, H. W. Longyear, a professor of gynecology and an abdominal surgeon in Detroit, published a book entitled *Nephrocoloptosis,* in which his main premise was that

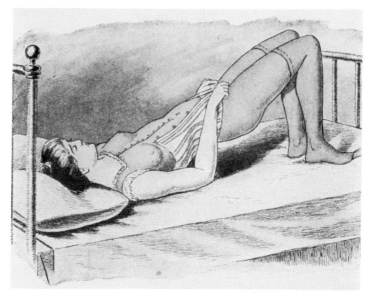

FIG. 51. *Corset for nephroptosis, demonstrating position for putting it on. (From Martin E, Thomas BA, Moorhead SW: White and Martin's Genito-Urinary Surgery and Venereal Diseases, 10th Ed, Philadelphia, Lippincott, 1918.)*

nephroptosis, unless traumatic, was secondary to enteroptosis. The nephrocolic ligament he described applied traction to the kidney in ptosis of the colon. His operation suspended first the colon and then the kidney.

Some surgeons such as Vogel, Albarran, and Narath actually used portions of the periostium and renal capsule to secure the kidney to the rib in the position desired. Others used slings of fascia to suspend the kidney (Figs. 52 and 53). These procedures slowly lost their popularity; at present, few of the younger urologists have seen or done nephropexy.

The term "focal infection" is usually applied to a local infection that produces symptoms in other parts of the body, without bacteria in the affected parts of the body and without bacteria in the blood. This was thought due to toxins in the

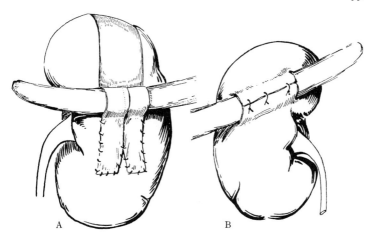

FIG. 52. *Nephropexies. A. After Vogel. B. After Narath. (From Israel J, Israel W: Chirurge der Niere and des Harnleiters. Leipzig, George Thieme, 1925.)*

circulation. In the years before bacteriostatic and antibiotic drugs, focal infection became an important part of medicine. For the sickly young person who couldn't gain weight and who had one illness or infection after another, focal infection was thought to be the source.

Rheumatic fever, infectious arthritis, chronic joint pains, recurrent headaches, and many other conditions were thought due to focal infections feeding toxins and organisms into the body. The tonsils, bad teeth, chronic appendicitis, and seminal vesiculitis were often considered the source. Seminal vesiculitis was one of the most frequently named sources of focal infection. Acute seminal vesiculitis differed from prostatitis in the rectal findings of enlarged vesicles and in symptoms of pain in the hip joint on the side or sides involved. Also, seminal vesiculitis was mistaken for acute appendicitis. Urethral discharge and digital findings on rectal examination should differentiate true seminal inflammation.

Therapy was directed at the vesicles through vasotomy with

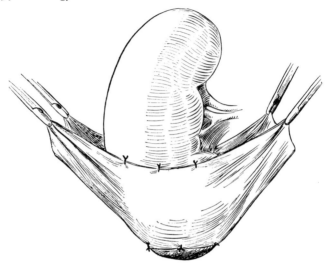

FIG. 53. *Suspension of the kidney in a hammock of fascia. (From Warbasse JP: Surgical Treatment. Philadelphia, WB Saunders, 1919.)*

the injection of therapeutic medications, incision, and drainage perineally of seminal vesicular abscess; even excision of the vesicles was often suggested and accomplished. Seminal vesicular cysts containing large amounts of fluid were often described in the older texts, but they are rarely found today. Seminal vesiculitis, although often named as the basis of hematospermia, is usually treated by neglect or prostate massage, or in some cases by mild antibacterial therapy over a long period. In the January 1931 issue of *Medical Clinics of North America*, Dr. Anson Clark, University of Pennsylvania, said:* "The close association that exists between tonsillar, dental and prostate infections is so constantly forced upon our notice that we naturally look in this direction for the answer."

* Clark Anson: Some experiences with recurrent dental infections and their influences upon infections of the urogenital tract. *Med Clin North Am 14:* 917–922, no. 4, 1931.

It was the consensus that prostatic infections were very common, secondary to infections elsewhere in the body. Focal infections also became much less important with the advent of chemotherapy.

In the late 1800s, seminal incontinence was considered so important a part of medical practice that there is an entire chapter so entitled in Pepper's *A System of Practical Medicine by American Authors.* In other books of the era there were large segments on this topic.*

By the term seminal incontinence; which is synonymous with involuntary or abnormal seminal emissions, pollutions and spermatorrhea, is meant the involuntary discharge of semen beyond the limits of health. Although usually described as a distinct disease, it is symptomatic of, and, as a rule, primarily dependent upon, weakness or exhaustion, along with exaggerated irritability, excitability, impressibility, or mobility of the centres which preside over erection and ejaculation.

Treatment varied tremendously, from setting an alarm clock for one hour before the time emissions generally occur, to sleeping on a hair mattress without much covering.

Everything calculated to induce a flow of blood to the genitalia, such as horseback exercise, driving over rough roads, and railway travelling, should be interdicted. Masturbation and sexual intercourse must be abandoned and the subject should be informed that the enforced rest of the organs will possibly result in temporary increased frequency of the pollutions. Chaste associations should be cultivated, and erotic thoughts and desires be banished.

In discussing this further it was said: ". . . attention is called to the fact that hyperesthesia of the prostatic urethra is nearly always present." In 1861, M. Lalleman wrote an entire book on this topic. *A Practical Treatise on the Causes, Symp-*

---

* Gross Samuel: Seminal incontinence. *A System of Practical Medicine by American Authors.* Vol IV, Edited by William Pepper. Philadelphia, Lea Brothers, 1886.

toms and Treatment of Spermatorrhoea was translated and went into many editions. He stated at the onset:*

During a period of fourteen years, I have collected more than one hundred and fifty cases in which involuntary seminal discharges were sufficiently serious to disorder the health of the patients considerably, and even some times to cause death. . . . a disease that degrades man, poisons the happiness of his best days, and ravages society.

This condition also has become less frequent and less well known. When such patients are seen today we search far and wide for the causes and generally give the all-encompassing diagnosis, "psychoneurotic." Prostatic massage, reassurance, and understanding are usually suggested therapies.

Prostatic atony as a cause of impotence was long considered important. Therapy for atony consisted of modalities aimed directly at the prostate. The psychrophore, a hollow metal finger-like instrument, was inserted in the rectum and cold water was run in and out, chilling the prostate and also the entire anus (Fig. 54). Electric diathermic insertions and warm water equipment were also used; some of these were utilized as well for prostatitis and seminal vesiculitis.

Vasectomy was advised at about the turn of the century to increase sexual potency. Usually it was done on one side only, but occasionally on both; the theory being to save all the male "juices" usually expended in orgasm and to recycle them into the body and make it stronger and more virile. The Steinach procedure was very popular. Monkey glands and goat glands were also big favorites for many years (see Chapter 13). Although prostatic atony as a diagnosis has fallen by the wayside, impotence has become more widespread, more important, and often less well handled.

Mercurochrome is another dead end of which many young

* Lalleman M: *A Practical Treatise on the Causes, Symptoms and Treatment of Spermatorrhoea.* 4th American Ed. Translated by Henry J McDougall. Philadelphia, Blanchard and Lea, 1861.

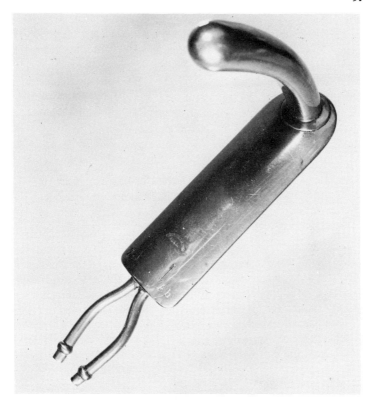

FIG. 54. *The psychrophore, used in the rectum for applying cold or warmth to the prostate in "prostatic atony." (Courtesy of the Urology Museum, The Albert Einstein College of Medicine, New York City.)*

physicians may not truly be aware. Invented at or shortly after the turn of the century, this drug was said to be able to do all the things that antibiotics later did. Hugh H. Young wrote a paper discussing its use in *JAMA* in 1919.* He showed that this mercurial could be used intravenously without coagulating albumin and otherwise "without toxicity." He found

* Young, HH: A new germicide for use in the genitourinary tract - mercurochrome 220. *JAMA* 73: 1483–1485, 1919.

blood and urine to be strongly bacteriostatic against *B. coli* with this therapy. Intravenous injections were followed by chills, fevers up to 106°, and other reactions including severe GI upsets. He reported unusual cures with this treatment. He also used intravenous gentian violet for staphylococcus infections.* Gentian violet injections are "immediately followed by a most alarming cyanosis, which is simply due to the dye in the blood, which causes no harm and passes off in a few hours." A markedly falling blood pressure and slowing of pulse are also sequelae that are not considered important. Cardiac stimulants are advised for "feeble patients."

It is a pleasure to quote Dr. Young again:

> In these cases we have the first demonstration that gentian violet may be used intravenously to combat general septicemia or local infections, and with remarkable success in the case of grampositive staphylococci. Coupled with the equally amazing results obtained with mercurochrome, these cases represent a splendid therapeutic achievement, and one is tempted to soar into realms of fancy and see a great variety of infectious processes treated and cured intravenously, but one must be restrained and cautious. Only by most careful study and painstaking selection and management of the cases can serious blunders be avoided, and it would not be safe as yet to risk not operating on certain fulminating infections that can now be cured by prompt surgery.

Another once-commonplace urologic activity that the modern urologist has not often seen is the syphilis clinic. At almost all general hospitals before the advent of penicillin there were large clinics given over to the diagnosis, treatment, and follow-up of lues veneria. Intravenous injections of arsenicals, alternating with courses of intramuscular injections of the heavy metals, usually mercury, were the rule and went on for months and years. These patients also had routine spinal taps in the OPD and spinal serologies were routine. Gummas, tabes, and

---

* Young HH: Treatment of septicemia and local infections by intravenous injections of mercurochrome 220 soluble and of gentian violet. *Trans South Surg Assn 36:* 515–540, 1924.

tertiary syphilis were often seen, as were hereditary syphilis and syphilis of the eyes, ears, and mouth. When penicillin became available, it was used at first in multiple-dose therapy and then in six-day continuous IV therapy; finally, we learned to use it as we do today.

Gonorrhea was treated with local therapy before antibiotics came on the scene. Anterior urethral injections of potassium permanganate were commonly used both therapeutically and prophylactically. The military establishment offered prophylactic stations where a soldier or sailor could get small tubes of a mercurial to inject intraurethrally, and also mercurials to rub into his penis and scrotum. He could first do an anterior irrigation with potassium permanganate and then use the mercurial in an attempt to prevent both syphilis and gonorrhea. If the anterior irrigation was too strenous, acute prostatitis often resulted.

Many instruments made their debut in urology over the years then faded into disuse as others more modern and better adapted to today's surgery were invented. Several instruments that disappeared with no replacements approximating their uses have long been forgotten. Zuckerkandl invented a corkscrew-like instrument to screw into the prostatic adenoma in order to be able to pull it from the fossa and bladder after enucleation (Fig. 55).

There was also a rabbit-eared hollow metal device containing chloroform-soaked cotton which was to be held in the hand of a patient undergoing cystoscopic examination (Fig. 56). The patient could insert the tips in his nostrils and inhale chloroform as desired to relieve his pain. When the patient became too deeply anesthetized, the hand and the instrument were supposed to fall away from the face. Later, a similar modern device using Trilene gas was marketed fairly unsuccessfully.

The Herman hook, with the appearance of a dock worker's instrument, was intended to pull specially cut catheters into the opened bladder to make a stab cystostomy. The instrument, clumsy as it was, worked. A long Kelly clamp worked

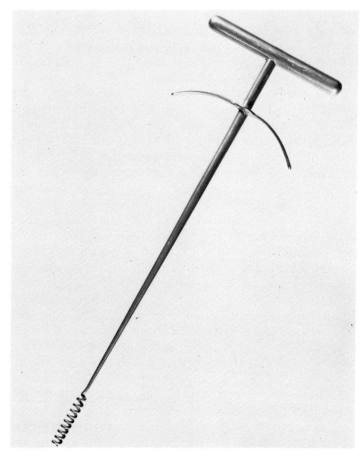

FIG. 55. *Zuckerkandl's prostatic extractor. (Courtesy of the Urology Museum, The Albert Einstein College of Medicine, New York City.)*

better however, and the Herman hook has disappeared with other useless instruments. Marcilles' net for ruptured kidneys has also been forgotten (Fig. 57).

A few of the other therapeutic modalities urologists used before the 1940s are worthy of mention. Before pyelography

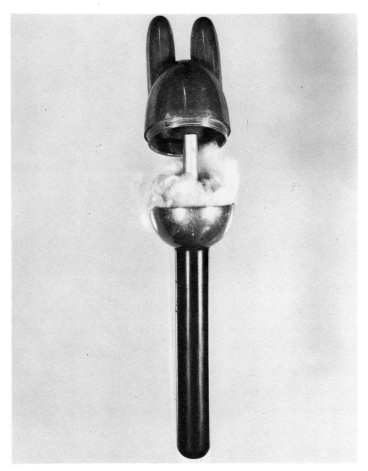

FIG. 56. *Self-anesthesia. With chloroform on the cotton, the two "ears" could be held to the nose; thus, the patient took a sniff when he desired. (Courtesy of the Urology Museum, The Albert Einstein College of Medicine, New York City.)*

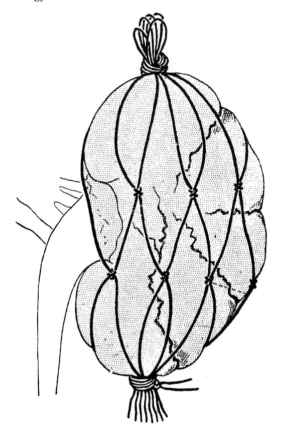

FIG. 57. *"Marcilles Net." Advised for multiple lacerations of the kidney. (From Albarran Joaquin: Operative Chirurgie der Harnwege. JENA, 1910.)*

was well developed, many urologists learned to make a smooth wax bulb on or near the tip of a urethral catheter. If the urologist was most careful in handling this, and could pass it up the ureter, contact with a calculus was supposed to result in a scratch on the otherwise smooth wax bulb, proving the diagnosis. Some urologists, after proving the presence of ureteral calculus and passing a catheter beyond it, instilled some sterile mineral oil or olive oil into the ureter or kidney above the stone. Theoretically this was to "oil the ureter" and ease the passage of the stone to the bladder. Some frightening renal reactions resulted. Rarely is this done in modern urology.

Urotropin was the drug of choice for most urinary infections in the years before antibiotics. This was straight methenamine and was the predecessor to Mandelamine. Not only was it the drug of choice, it was for many years practically the only drug.

Neosalvarsan, an arsenical antisyphilitic drug, was used sometimes for severe or acute pyelonephritis with good results. Typhoid vaccine, with a severe febrile reaction for 24 to 48 hours, was sometimes effective against severe systemic infections such as acute gonorrheal arthritis.

Urethritis, acute or chronic, was treated in many ways. Some of the therapies no longer in favor with urologists are Argyrol instillations and the "sealing–in" therapy with Argyrol as described in 1939 by Leon Herman:*

Sealing–in treatment of gonorrhea is often used with the idea of aborting the disease. The method is as follows: With the patient lying prone, a thick strip of cotton is wound around the base of the penis in such manner that the organ is held upright. About 3 cc. of freshly prepared Argyrol solution (5 per cent) is injected into the anterior urethra. The glans is thoroughly dried. Then several drops of flexible collodion are placed on the cotton-covered meatus, more of the collodion is added (drop by drop) until a cap is formed over the anterior portion of the glans. The Argyrol is retained for six or eight hours if possible. The patient is instructed to drink sparingly of water, and to empty the bladder just before the injection of the Argyrol. For removal of the cap, he is instructed to immerse the penis in warm water. The treatment is repeated once or twice daily. . . . Our records show a number cured after one week's treatment.

Posterior instillations were very frequently administered by urologists using the Guyon instillator. This was similar to a

* Herman Leon: *Practise of Urology*. Philadelphia, WB Saunders, 1939.

shortened male silver catheter that could be used with a syringe. Silver nitrate or Argyrol or other materials were deposited with this instrument into the seat of infection, the posterior urethra. Acriflavine, a dye, was the favorite of many urologists for instillation and irrigations.

Many other therapeutic modalities have, of course, disappeared from use. Many instruments no longer are manufactured; many drugs are no longer available. Modern methods have made them obsolete.

Bibliography

There is no way that I can list all the books, articles, lectures, and discussions that have been used as background material for this volume. To help those interested in reading further, I have listed a few titles for each topic, and then only the ones that I have enjoyed or found especially helpful. This should in no way be confused with a complete bibliography. It is merely a list of references I think might enhance the reader's enjoyment.

BOOKS ABOUT THE HISTORY OF MEDICINE OR UROLOGY

Bhishagratna KL: An English translation of the *Sushruta Samhita*. Varanasi, India, Chowkhamba Sanskrit Series Office, 1963.
Very interesting, but covers a lot of territory. Excellent on aphrodisiacs and lithotomy.

Bitschai J, and Brodny ML: *A History of Urology in Egypt*. New York City, Riverside Press, 1956.
Good reading; a valuable short book. Helps in visualizing ancient Egypt.

Dana Charles L: *The Peaks of Medical History*. New York City, Hoeber, 1926.
Those periods discussed are well done; not much urology, however.

165

Garrison Fielding H: *An Introduction to the History of Medicine.* 4th Ed, WB Saunders, Philadelphia, 1929.
Well-written, crammed with names and facts, a good source book.

Gordon BL: *Medicine Throughout Antiquity.* Philadelphia, FA Davis, 1949.
Easily read; good illustrations.

Levey M: *The Medical Formulary or Aqrābādhīn of al-Kindī* (trans). Madison, University of Wisconsin Press, 1966.
Presents a facet rarely commented on in most histories.

Lewis Bransford (ed): *History of Urology* (under the auspices of the American Urological Assoc.). Baltimore, Williams & Wilkins, 1933.
These two volumes are a good source from which to research the development of urology. Written by many urologists; on the whole not very exciting.

Murphy LJT: *The History of Urology.* Springfield, Charles C. Thomas, 1972. Published since this book was written, it combines a translated History of Urology from Desnos' Encyclopedia francais with Murphy's own modernization in the second part. Fine reading and excellent history.

Pousson A, Desnos E (eds): *Encyclopédie francaise d'urologie.* Paris, Octave Doin et Fils, 1914–1923.
This six volume enyclopedia is amazingly interesting. Desnos alone has written some 294 pages in review of the development of urology. Even if you can't read French, it's still very worthwhile if only for the numerous illustrations in color and in black and white.

Renouard PV: *History of Medicine* (trans). Philadelphia, Lindsay & Blakiston, 1867.
A big book covering all of medicine; not very valuable urologically, except as it fits into the entire picture of the development of medicine.

Sigerist HE: *A History of Medicine.* Vol I: *Primitive and Archaic Medicine,* 1951; Vol. II: *Early Greek, Hindu, and Persian Medicine,* 1961. New York City, Oxford University Press.
Written interestingly; both enjoyable and educational, something rare.

Veith Ilza (ed and trans): *Huang-Ti Nei-Ching Su-Wên* (The Yellow Emperor's Classic of Internal Medicine). University of Berkeley, California Press, 1966.
If you can wade through it, there is much of interest.

Watson J: *The Medical Profession in Ancient Times.* New York City, Baker & Godwin, 1856.
Pictures ancient Roman and Greek times and the physicians who made the science famous.

GOOD TEXTS ON UROLOGY BEFORE 1930

Albarran J: *Operative Chirurgie der Harnwege.* Jena, Fischer, 1910.
An excellent picture of early twentieth century urology. In German.

Chetwood Charles H: *The Practice of Urology.* New York City, William Wood, 1916.
An 825-page book, easily followed. Urology before World War I; well illustrated.

Guyon JCF: *Leçons cliniques sur les maladies de voies urinaires.* Paris, 1881.
Few illustrations; two volumes.

Martin E, Thomas BA, Moorhead SW: *White and Martin's Genito-Urinary Surgery and Venereal Diseases.* Philadelphia, Lippincott. (Many editions—mine was the tenth in 1917).
This book was the bible for many urologists up to and including World War I. VD was much more important to the urologist then.

Van Buren WH, and Keyes EL: *A Practical Treatise on the Surgical Diseases of the Genito-Urinary Organs, Including Syphilis.* New York City, Appleton, 1876.
Cases and good illustrations included. Designed as a manual for students and practitioners. The forerunner to Keyes' famous texts in 1918 and thereafter.

Wildbolz Hans: *Lehrbuch der Urologie.* Berlin, Springer, 1924.
Good illustrations.

Young Hugh H: *Young's Practice of Urology.* Philadelphia, WB Saunders, 1926.
A classic text far in advance of its time, based on a study of 12,500 cases. Beautifully and profusely illustrated.

VENEREAL DISEASES

Bell Benjamin: *A Treatise on Gonorrhoea Virulenta and Lues Venerea.* Philadelphia, Robert Campbell, 1795.
Discusses the possibility that poorly treated gonorrhea might turn into pox (syphilis). Discusses strictures, hemorrhages, gleets, and swelling of the testicles, cords, and glands. Good discussion of mercury therapy and its consequences; also important for strictures.

Buchan W: *Observations Concerning the Prevention and Cure of the Venereal Disease.* London, Chapman, 1796.

Bumstead FJ (ed and trans) : *A Treatise on the Venereal Disease* (by John Hunter with additions by Philippe Ricord). 2nd Ed, Philadelphia, Blanchard & Lea, 1859.
A fascinating book; opposing ideas placed together.

Ricord Philippe: *Traité pratique des maladies vénériennes.* Paris, 1838.
The man who did experimental work on inoculations of lues and gonorrhea.

Schwediauer FX: *Practical Observations on Obstinate and Inveterate Venereal Complaints.* London, Johnson, 1784.
"The author of the following small treatise has made it his business to examine all that has been written on the veneral disease. . . ." Well-written, enjoyable.

PROSTATE AND URINARY RETENTION

Freyer PJ: *Clinical Lectures on Enlargement of the Prostate* with a description of the author's operation of total enucleation of the Organ. 3rd Ed, New York City, William Wood, 1906.
Suprapubic prostatectomy described by the author who claimed priority. Nicely illustrated.

Petit A (ed) : *Amussat's Lectures on Retention of Urine* (trans). Philadelphia, Haswell, Barrington & Haswell, 1840.
Interesting illustrations of the problems of the period, when surgery was just beginning to assume a place in medical science.

Pilcher PM: *Transvesical Prostatectomy in Two Stages.* Philadelphia, Lippincott, 1914.
Argues the anatomy and pathology, and describes the surgery.

Weldon Walter: *Observations on the Different Modes of the Puncturing of the Bladder, in Cases of Retention of Urine.* Southampton, London, Printed by T Baker for W Dawson, 1793.

CYSTOSCOPE AND TUR

Casper Leopold: *Lehrbuch der Urologie.* Berlin, Urban & Schwarzenberg, 1923.

Kelly HA, Ward GE: *Electrosurgery.* Philadelphia, WB Saunders, 1932.
.Well-illustrated. Describes the beginnings; not limited to GU tract.

Fenwick EH: *The Electric Illumination of the Bladder and Urethra.* London, J&A Churchill, 1889.
Excellent illustrations of early instrumentation and case histories.

Luys Georges: *A Treatise on Cystoscopy and Urethroscopy* (trans).
St. Louis, Mosby, 1918.
Profusely illustrated for instrumental development and clinical findings.

Kidney

Simon Gustav: *Chirurgie der Nieren.* Erlangen, 1871.
By the first man to do a nephrectomy.

Bladder Tumors

Beer Edwin: *Tumors of the Urinary Bladder.* Baltimore, William Wood, 1935.
Good historical sketch, well-illustrated; 166 pages of interest.

Urinalysis

Fletcher: The Differences, Causes and Judgments of Urine Analysis. Lecture memoranda AMA, London, Burroughs Wellcome & Co, 1911. *An Historical Sketch of the Clinical Examination of Urine* is the subtitle.
A nicely done, well-illustrated little book covering the entire story up to that time.

Dahl Ludvig: *Heller's Pathological Chemistry of the Urine.* Dublin, Fannin, 1855.
A small handbook. It also contains chapters on blood, milk, vomitus, and feces. Discusses urophaein, uroxanthin, uric acid, and hippuric acid.

Flint Austin, Jr: *Manual of Chemical Examination of the Urine in Disease.* New York City, Appleton, 1870.
This is the classic "pocket-book" for the medical practitioner.

Stricture and Urethra

Bell Charles: *Letters Concerning the Diseases of the Urethra.* London, Printed for John Murray in Fleet Street. Edinburgh, Bell and Bradfeete, 1810.

Segalas PS: *De la Cautérisation des Ritrecissements Organiques de l'urethre.* Paris, 1829.

Thompson Henry: *The Pathology and Treatment of Stricture of the Urethra and Urinary Fistulae.* Philadelphia, Henry C Lea, 1869.
These three interesting volumes show the severity of the problem of stricture in the 1800s.

Lithotomy and Stone Disease

Bigelow Henry J: *Litholapaxy or Rapid Lithotrity with Evacuation.* Boston, A Williams, 1878.
A classic of its time, litholapaxy and its instrumentation first described.

Civiale Jean: *Lettres sur la Lithotritie or L'Art de Broyer la Pierre.* Paris, 1837.

Civiale Jean: *Medical and Prophylactic Treatment of Stone and Gravel* (trans). Philadelphia, Waldie, 1841.
These two books are by one of the French pioneers in the treatment of bladder stones. Interesting concepts of lithogenesis and therapy.

d'Étiolles Leroy: *De la Lithotripsie.* Paris, Bailliere, 1836.
By the man who did so much to advance the science of breaking stones.

Ellis Harold: *A History of Bladder Stone.* Oxford, England, Blackwell, 1969.
A profusely illustrated, easily read story.

Falconer William: *An Account of the Efficacy of the Aqua Mephitica Alkalina or Solution of Fixed Alkaline Salt, Saturated with Fixible Air in Calculous Disorders and Other Complaints of the Urinary Passages.* London, 1789.
Many interesting case reports.

Lobb Theophilus: *Treatise on Dissolvents of the Stone and on Curing the Stone and Gout by Aliment.* London, Buckland, 1739.
Very interesting. Rules of diet, probabilities of dissolving stones in the kidney or bladder. Experiments discussed and cases presented.

Rutty John: *An Account of Some New Experiments and Observations on Joanna Stephens' Medicine for the Stone.* London, printed for R Mausky, over against the old Bailey on Ludgate hill, 1742.
Very interesting presentation to the Royal Society, excellent introductory remarks by the author. Cases and results.

Snip F: *Dissertatio de Lithotomia.* Amsterdam, Schrueder, 1761.
In Latin, a beautiful little book, no illustrations.

Tolet F: *Traité de la Lithotomie.* 4th Ed, Paris, 1689.
In French, excellent illustrations, a pleasure to read.

SOME INTERESTING BOOKS

Armstrong John W: *The Water of Life—A Treatise on Urine Therapy.* 2nd Ed, London, True Health Publishing Co, 1944.
Treats gangrene, cancer, leukemia, heart disease, and venereal disease. Interesting concept used by the ancients before Christ.

Davenport John: *Aphrodisiacs and Anti-Aphrodisiacs.* London, 1869.
Three essays on the powers of reproduction. Covers the ancients, phallic worship, impotence, and aphrodisiacs. Well-written and illustrated.

Voronoff Serge, Alexandrescu George: *Testicular Grafting from Ape to Man, Operative Technique, Physiological Manifestations,*

Histological Evolution and Statistics (trans). London, Brentano, 1923.

ARTICLES WORTH LOOKING AT

Buerger Leo: A historical survey of the development of modern urological instruments. *Urol Cutan Rev* 35:1–25, 1931.
An excellent article.

Murphy Leonard JT: The art of uroscopy. *Med J Aust* 2:879–886, 1967.

Riches Eric: The history of lithotomy and lithotrity. *Ann Roy Coll Surg Eng* 43:185–199, 1968.

INDEX

Cover design by Patrick H. Turner

73 74 75 76 77 78 10 9 8 7 6 5 4 3 2 1